PCOS Weight Loss Diet Plan

This Guide Will Help Reverse PCOS Fertility Issues

Karie Milstein

© Copyright 2020 - All rights reserved.

The content contained within this book may not be reproduced, duplicated or transmitted without direct written permission from the author or the publisher.

Under no circumstances will any blame or legal responsibility be held against the publisher, or author, for any damages, reparation, or monetary loss due to the information contained within this book, either directly or indirectly.

Legal Notice:

This book is copyright protected. It is only for personal use. You cannot amend, distribute, sell, use, quote or paraphrase any part, or the content within this book, without the consent of the author or publisher.

Disclaimer Notice:

Please note the information contained within this document is for educational and entertainment purposes only. All effort has been executed to present accurate, up to date, reliable, complete information. No warranties of any kind are declared or implied. Readers acknowledge that the author is not engaged in the rendering of legal, financial, medical or professional advice. The content within this book has been derived from various sources. Please consult a licensed professional before attempting any techniques outlined in this book.

By reading this document, the reader agrees that under no circumstances is the author responsible for any losses, direct or indirect, that are incurred as a result of the use of the information contained within this document, including, but not limited to, errors, omissions, or inaccuracies.

Table of Contents

INTRODUCTION 1
   A Brief Overview 3

CHAPTER 1: DIAGNOSED WITH PCOS? 7
   What to Look For 11
      Hirsutism 12
      Hair Loss 12
      Fatigue 13
      Mood Swings 14
      Migraines 14
      Sugar Cravings 15
      Weight Gain 15
      Acne 16
      Fertility Issues 16
   How PCOS is Diagnosed 16
   What to Do After You Have Been Diagnosed 18
      Educate Yourself 19
      Assemble a Top-Notch Team 20
      Get Support 22
      Observe Your Body 23
      Be Kind to Yourself 24
   Questions to Ask Your Doctor 26
      Do I Need to Take Birth Control Pills? 27
      How Can I Lower Risk of Complications? 28
      How Will PCOS Affect My Fertility? 28

CHAPTER 2: ALL ABOUT PCOS 31
   What is PCOS? 31
   Symptoms of PCOS 34
      Triad of Symptoms 35
      Symptoms for Diagnosis 37

- CAUSES OF PCOS 38
- TREATMENTS FOR PCOS 40
  - *Prescribed Treatments*... 41
  - *Natural Treatments* 46
- POSSIBLE COMPLICATIONS OF PCOS SYMPTOMS 49
  - *Infertility* 50
  - *Bloating* 51
  - *Uterine Bleeding* 51
  - *Diabetes*.. 52
  - *High Blood Pressure*.. 53
  - *High Cholesterol* 55
  - *Sleep Apnea* 56
  - *Depression and Anxiety* 58
  - *Endometrial Cancer* 61
  - *Nonalcoholic Steatohepatitis*.. 63
  - *Metabolic Syndrome*.. 64
- EFFECTS ON PREGNANCY 65
  - *Miscarriage*... 66
  - *Pregnancy-Induced High Blood Pressure* 67
  - *Gestational Diabetes* 68
  - *Preeclampsia* 69
  - *Preterm Birth* 72
  - *Cesarean Delivery*... 72
  - *Fetal Macrosomia*.. 73
- MYTHS ABOUT PCOS 75
  - *PCOS is a Rare Condition* 76
  - *You Did Something to Cause PCOS* 76
  - *You Cannot Get Pregnant If You Have PCOS* 77
  - *PCOS Symptoms End at Menopause* 77
  - *Losing Weight Stops PCOS Symptoms* 79

CHAPTER 3: YOUR WEIGHT AND PCOS 81

- WEIGHT AND PCOS 83
- WEIGHT LOSS.. 85
  - *Cardio* 85
  - *Weight Training*... 88
  - *Yoga*.. 88
- WHY IT IS HARD TO LOSE WEIGHT WITH PCOS 99

CHAPTER 4: CHANGING YOUR LIFESTYLE FOR PCOS 103

- MANAGING PCOS WITH LIFESTYLE 104
  - *Physical Activity* *105*
  - *Food* *109*
  - *Sleep* *113*
- PRACTICE SELF-CARE 121
  - *Reduce Stress* *122*
  - *Clear Mental Roadblocks* *128*
  - *Overcome Challenges* *131*
- AVOID ENDOCRINE DISRUPTORS 132

CHAPTER 5: YOUR PCOS DIET 137

- WHAT TO ADD TO OR REMOVE FROM YOUR DIET 138
  - *Foods to Add* *138*
  - *Foods to Remove* *142*
- THREE DIETS THAT MAY HELP PEOPLE WITH PCOS 145
  - *Anti-Inflammatory Diet* *145*
  - *Low Glycemic Index Diet* *150*
  - *Dietary Approaches to Stop Hypertension (DASH) Diet.* *155*
- NUTRIENTS TO INCREASE 161
  - *Vitamin D and Calcium* *162*
  - *Iron* *163*
  - *Magnesium* *164*
  - *Chromium* *165*
  - *Omega-3s* *165*
  - *Zinc* *166*
- OTHER TIPS 167
- MEAL AND SNACK SUGGESTIONS 169
  - *Breakfast* *169*
  - *Lunch* *173*
  - *Dinner* *177*
  - *Snacks* *182*
  - *Sample Meal Plan Menus* *185*
  - *Flavor Tips* *188*

CHAPTER 6: BOOSTING YOUR FERTILITY 191

- LIFESTYLE CHANGES 193

- MEDICATION 196
  - *Oral Medications* *196*
  - *Injected Hormones* *197*
- ASSISTED REPRODUCTIVE TECHNOLOGIES 199
  - *Intrauterine Insemination (IUI)* *200*
  - *In vitro Fertilization* *200*
  - *Gamete Intrafallopian Transfer* *201*
- SURGICAL OPTIONS 201
  - *Ovarian Drilling* *202*
  - *Hysteroscopic Surgery* *202*
  - *Tubal Surgery* *203*

CHAPTER 7: MANAGING YOUR PCOS SYMPTOMS 205

- HIRSUTISM 205
- HAIR LOSS 207
- ACNE 209
- OTHER SKIN ISSUES 211
- MENTAL HEALTH ISSUES 213
- EMOTIONAL HEALTH CARE 215

CONCLUSION 219

REFERENCES 223

"Natural forces within us are the true healers of disease."

by Hippocrates

Introduction

Would you believe that there is a disorder that affects up to ten percent of women worldwide, gets progressively worse over time, and takes years on average to be diagnosed (Rao et al., 2020)? The United States spends almost $4 billion a year diagnosing and helping women treat symptoms of this disorder (*30 Interesting Facts About PCOS*, 2017). It sounds far-fetched, like it must be a condition everyone has heard of, something for which charities passionately raise funding, a disorder with its own marathon and catchy slogan.

It is Polycystic Ovary Syndrome, or PCOS. Have you heard of it? Are you suffering from it? Did it take years to get a diagnosis? Are you still waiting to find relief from your symptoms?

My name is Karie Milstein, and I wrote this book because I wish something like it had been available for me years ago. I was diagnosed with PCOS when I was a teenager. I was overweight and suffering from cystic acne, but my doctor could not figure out what was causing my discomfort. It took a while for us to put all of the pieces together and pinpoint PCOS as the disorder. I started to do my own research, determined to control my condition without medication. Over the years I changed my diet, lost fifty pounds, and managed to have a baby without any medical intervention.

I want to share what I learned from my own experiences and from over five years of extensive PCOS research. I love studying hormonal balance and how it affects women's health. While doing my research, I have met and interviewed many women who have struggled with PCOS symptoms. Everyone's experience is different, as you will see here. Many stories I will be sharing have common threads of shared symptoms like weight gain, irregular periods, excess hair growth, and more, but some stories are different. You may be experiencing common symptoms, or you may be experiencing something that seems to have come out of left field. No matter what symptoms you are struggling with, reading about what other women have gone through will help you realize you can harness the strength to manage this condition.

I have experienced what you are experiencing in terms of symptoms and the struggle to get a diagnosis, and I can help you because I have been through this pain. Living with PCOS is a never-ending journey, but it does not have to be a struggle. I can help you achieve a healthy lifestyle so you can keep your PCOS symptoms in check and learn to love your body again.

A Brief Overview

PCOS is the most common hormonal condition that affects women of reproductive age. Symptoms typically present around a woman's first menstrual cycle, but can appear later and often become more severe over time. Research shows that while one in ten women have PCOS, only half of them know it. PCOS affects women physically, mentally, and reproductively.

While the exact cause of PCOS is unknown, genetics possibly play a part. One theory is that excess insulin can cause PCOS. When your body produces excess insulin, you build up a resistance. This resistance can raise your blood sugar levels while also increasing androgen production that complicates ovulation.

Another theory of the cause of PCOS is high levels of androgen. Androgen is commonly referred to as a "male hormone," though all women have some in small amounts. Having a high level of androgen causes acne, male pattern baldness, and extra hair growth in other places, like facial hair or body hair. All of these are symptoms of PCOS. Too much androgen can also prevent a woman's ovaries from releasing eggs during her menstrual cycles (*Polycystic ovary syndrome | Womenshealth.gov*, 2019).

There is no cure for PCOS, but being diagnosed early can help prevent further complications like diabetes and heart disease. Lifestyle changes such as a healthy diet and weight loss can help keep PCOS symptoms manageable.

After your diagnosis, you will want to educate yourself, and this book is an excellent way to do that. While you will find plenty of research, helpful tips, and diet suggestions, you will still want to make sure you have a solid support team. These can be friends and family in real life, or through online support groups. Living with PCOS can be rough, and for those days when you feel like you cannot make it through, you will want to have some cheerleaders inspiring you to get out of bed and do your best.

We will go over the symptoms and the possible treatments available to you. Your doctor may go over some of these with you, but it is always a good idea to research on your own. While it is nice to think that your doctor has your best interests at heart, unfortunately that is not always the case. It is best to know your options and choose something that will work best for your lifestyle, your body, and your mental health.

PCOS is a serious disorder, and there are complications if you let it go untreated. However, some of the information you will hear about PCOS are myths, so you will learn the truth about these before we delve too deeply into everything.

Managing your weight is a priority when it comes to living with PCOS, but if you change your lifestyle, improve your diet, and add in some physical activity, that task will be easier than you might think. Even practicing self-care and giving yourself the grace to overcome daily challenges will lessen the stress you feel, which can exacerbate PCOS.

There are three diets that can help you manage your PCOS and lose weight, but even if you do not follow these diets by the book, you will learn what nutrients can help you stay healthy, along with suggestions for meals and snacks.

You can boost your fertility in many ways, and we will explore them all, whether it is naturally, using medical procedures, assisted reproductive technology, or researching surgical options.

I will walk you through all of the steps I took to get all aspects of my condition under control. I know everyone is different, even if we have all been diagnosed with the same disorder. We will be exploring plenty of options so you are sure to find something that works for you and your body.

Chapter 1:

Diagnosed with PCOS?

Most women with PCOS experience years of being shuffled between doctors before they are given a diagnosis. The women's stories shared here were shared on a public forum, but names have been changed to keep them anonymous.

Kelly first got her period when she was eleven, and it was irregular for years. She would have a period six to ten times a year; sometimes it was light, and sometimes it was incredibly heavy, literally lasting for months. Her doctor told her it was because she played sports and had an athletic build. Kelly's doctor prescribed pills to help make her periods more regular.

When Kelly started college, she started gaining weight. She figured it was because she was on her own for the first time, eating more junk food than ever before, while being less active than she used to be. Besides, it seems everyone gained the Freshman Fifteen. But Kelly gained more than fifteen pounds, and she started to notice hair on her face where she had not had any before.

The next time Kelly visited her doctor, she was very vocal about how uncomfortable she felt in her body and that she was sure something was wrong. The doctor took an ultrasound of Kelly's ovaries and found she had multiple cysts. Further testing showed that Kelly was insulin resistant. But none of that mattered much to Kelly—she heard that there was no cure and felt defeated.

Three other women shared stories similar to Kelly's, with a few minor details that were different. One woman had been overweight since childhood, and one had not experienced a standard growth spurt that thinned her out before reaching puberty. Another woman did not gain weight at all, but had irregular periods and excessive body hair.

One woman told a story that had different symptoms, such as a sensitivity to sugar and excessive sweating. These are symptoms of PCOS that often are not initially linked to the disorder, but that does not make them any less common, or any easier to endure. The sensitivity to sugar is linked to the insulin resistance thought to be a cause of PCOS. However, problems with insulin can be a symptom of many diseases, so it is often not immediately linked to PCOS. Doctors might run tests relating to diabetes or cardiovascular problems, and when those come back clear, not know where to go from there.

In all of these cases, it took years of doctor's visits before they were diagnosed with PCOS. Some doctors do not think that the women are really suffering from any of the symptoms they claim, and the women struggle with finding a specialist who will believe them and advocate for them. Too often a doctor does not connect the symptoms and relate them to the larger problem of PCOS. This typically happens when young women experience symptoms while going through puberty and being relatively new to menstrual cycles. Since the women are new to periods and are experiencing various bodily changes, doctors might write off any concerns as just being something with which the women are unfamiliar. Doctors think things will work out as the woman's body develops, so the condition is written off as being isolated symptoms that will level out in time. Some women only see their doctor for annual checkups, so it is easy to see how it takes years for PCOS to be diagnosed.

Amanda had been struggling with her weight for years before she realized there might be a bigger issue at hand. Overweight women who go to their doctors with other PCOS symptoms are often told to lose weight first, as if that is a cure-all. While weight loss can help manage PCOS symptoms, it should not be an alternative to other testing options. Weight gain can be a symptom of PCOS more than the cause, and doctors might not be sensitive to that issue.

Amanda was frustrated that her doctor saw her weight as causing all of the other symptoms she was experiencing, instead of the larger problem actually causing her weight gain. She felt blamed for her struggle, and that caused her mental health to suffer, which only exacerbated her other symptoms. Once she was diagnosed, Amanda and her doctor were able to work together to manage her PCOS symptoms, and her doctor stopped treating weight loss like a magical cure-all.

Sarah has a different story from women who suffered since puberty; she had no complications until, in her early 20s, she missed a period. She went to her gynecologist, who took an ultrasound and diagnosed Sarah with PCOS. Her doctor almost laughed it off, Sarah remembers, still angry. Sarah's doctor said that many women would love to not have a period, and that Sarah should not worry about it until she was trying to conceive. But it is not that easy to brush off a condition that affects your entire well-being.

Though Sarah's doctor displayed a levity that Sarah herself could not feel, it helped that she did not experience symptoms until she was older. Sarah already had a history with her gynecologist so it was easier to detect that something was wrong. Of course, it helps that Sarah's doctor was a specialist who knew to look for such things.

Many women's stories have that common thread—their regular doctors were relatively calm about symptoms they were experiencing, and were not able to make the connection to PCOS until it had persisted for years. On the other hand, gynecologists typically made the connection immediately.

Some women do not realize that what they are experiencing is not just how their body is meant to be.

PCOS and menstruation or reproductive issues are not common topics of conversation, so a woman feeling pain during her period might not know it should not be that way. Women might not feel comfortable sharing their symptoms with a doctor, or if they get brushed off once, they might not think it is worth bringing up the topic again.

Every woman interviewed stressed the same point: be outspoken. Be your own advocate. A doctor might not intend to disregard your input, but it happens too often. Do your own research and come to your appointments informed. Do not be afraid to ask for certain tests or scans. Even if you are tested for various symptoms and the results come back with no definitive diagnosis, keep pushing for answers. It might take time to put all of the pieces together, but you know your body better than anyone else. If something does not feel right, keep seeking a solution.

If your advocacy does lead to a diagnosis, then you have taken one step forward to taking control of this condition, instead of letting it control you.

What to Look For

If you think you are suffering from PCOS, there are some symptoms that could help you understand before you are diagnosed. These symptoms are not exclusive to PCOS, so even if you are experiencing many or all of them, that is not a definite diagnosis. You always need to check with your doctor before jumping to conclusions, but it is a great idea to be educated before your appointment.

Hirsutism

Hirsutism is excessive hair growth in women due to high levels of androgen. Where women might typically have "peach fuzz," like on their face, hirsutism causes that hair to grow in dark and coarse. Over seventy-five percent of women with hirsutism have PCOS, but not everyone diagnosed with PCOS will have hirsutism (Yildiz et al., 2010). This can also be a symptom of other disorders, like a thyroid disease.

Hair Loss

Hair loss can be called female androgenic alopecia or female pattern hair loss, which is caused by high levels of androgen, a symptom of PCOS. Unlike male pattern baldness, female pattern hair loss is just a thinning of the hair at the top of your head and around the hairline. The follicles do not die, so your hair can still grow back.

As previously mentioned, hair loss alone is not an indication that you have PCOS. Other conditions that can cause hair loss are menopause, anemia, thyroid conditions, or an autoimmune disease. Thinning hair and hair loss can also be side effects of medication, so it is important to take all of this into consideration when you talk to your doctor.

Fatigue

Fatigue is a symptom of PCOS, but it is also a symptom of many other conditions. Your everyday life can also cause fatigue, so you should only consider this a symptom if you are feeling it to an extreme degree you have never felt before, and in tandem with other symptoms from this list.

If you are feeling fatigued, first try to handle it yourself. Make sure you are prioritizing rest, whether it is taking naps during the day, getting a full night's sleep, or even just lessening your stress load. Eating a more nutritious diet can also help decrease your feelings of fatigue.

Fatigue can also be a side effect of some medications. It can also be a symptom of other disorders, like anemia, diabetes, fibromyalgia, sleep disorders, or autoimmune diseases. Be honest with your doctor about the type of fatigue you feel—does it take you a while to wake up in the morning, or are you dragging all day? Try to think of things that might be triggering your fatigue, like if you are tired after eating certain foods or doing certain activities. Being able to pinpoint the cause of your fatigue will help your doctor figure out if it is related to PCOS or not.

Mood Swings

It is normal to have mood swings, especially around your period or when you are ovulating, due to a disruption in your hormones. If not related to hormones, mood swings can be associated with anxiety and depression, which can also be linked to PCOS. Just as you should pinpoint the cause of your fatigue, try to do this with your mood swings before you see your doctor. Knowing that your mood swings seem unrelated to your menstrual cycle or something more common like work stress will help your doctor factor it into your diagnosis.

Having mood swings if you are not having a regular period is also a sign pointing to PCOS. If you are not having a regular period and not ovulating regularly yet still having mood swings, you could possibly have PCOS. But since they are also linked to anxiety and depression, you should be aware of your mood swings and seek help for them regardless of if they are part of PCOS or not. Your mental health is just as important as your physical health.

Migraines

Migraines are not specifically linked to PCOS, but many accounts women have shared about PCOS symptoms have included migraines. They are especially alarming if you have never had them before, but start experiencing them along with any of the other symptoms on this list.

Sugar Cravings

Because a possible cause of PCOS is insulin resistance, craving sugar all of the time is a symptom. Women diagnosed with PCOS have high insulin levels, which inhibits their appetite-regulating hormones, so they feel hungrier more often. While sugar and carbs might satiate that hunger, they are not healthy options and will lead to weight gain.

If you are experiencing excessive sugar cravings, try to eat healthy options instead of giving in to the craving. If you make healthy choices and stop feeling these cravings, tell your doctor so that can be taken into consideration for your diagnosis.

Weight Gain

Due to insulin resistance, it is easy to gain weight when you have PCOS. Many women have reported excessive weight gain as one of the signs they knew something was wrong with their bodies. While sometimes this gain relates to the previously mentioned sugar cravings, it often is your body's resistance to insulin that makes your body store fat. This resistance makes it difficult to lose weight once you have put it on.

Acne

Along with higher levels of androgen, women with PCOS have higher levels of testosterone. This hormone causes acne that will make you feel like you are a teenager again, but not in a good way! Breakouts are not solely associated with PCOS, though; it can also be a symptom of other hormone fluctuations, stress, or reactions to topical products.

Fertility Issues

If you have been trying to get pregnant but are struggling, you might have fertility issues caused by PCOS. The condition interferes with your menstrual cycles and ovulation, which can make it hard to get pregnant. Having problems with fertility does not mean you have PCOS, though. Family history, age, weight, and thyroid conditions can also play a part in infertility.

How PCOS is Diagnosed

It is rare for two women to experience the same symptoms, so it is important to be aware of all of the possible symptoms associated with PCOS. If you feel like you are experiencing symptoms that could be related to PCOS, make an appointment with your healthcare provider. There is no specific test that will diagnose you with PCOS, but a variety of tests can help you and your doctor gain a deeper understanding of what you are experiencing and why.

Your healthcare provider will ask you questions about your medical history, including your menstrual cycles and weight changes, as well as your specific symptoms. They will give you a physical exam to check for any excess hair or acne. The physical exam should include a pelvic exam, even if the symptoms you have experienced have not yet had anything to do with your menstrual cycle. The pelvic exam will give your doctor an opportunity to check for any growths or abnormalities in your reproductive organs.

Your doctor should also conduct an ultrasound. This will help them see the size of your ovaries. If you have cysts on your ovaries, they will be visible on the ultrasound. Cysts are fluid-filled sacs that form in the ovaries, but you can be diagnosed with PCOS without having cysts.

The ultrasound will also gauge your endometrium—the mucus membrane that lines your uterus. This membrane gets thicker during your menstrual cycle to be ready for embryo implantation. In some instances, women will not ovulate because of a lack of hormones. This is what may cause your period to be irregular. A lack of ovulation can also cause cysts to form on your ovaries, though again, not all women who have PCOS have cysts.

You will also go through blood tests, which can detect high levels of androgen, the "male hormone" that causes excessive hair growth in women with PCOS. Blood tests will also track the levels of glucose, cholesterol, and triglyceride. If you have a resistance to insulin, this can be determined through blood tests (*Polycystic Ovary Syndrome (PCOS)*, 2019).

Doctors typically make a diagnosis if two out of three criteria are met. These include:

- High levels of androgens are found in your blood
- Ovaries have partly formed eggs, or the size of one or both ovaries is increased
- You have a lack of menstrual periods, experience irregular cycles, or do not ovulate.

What to Do After You Have Been Diagnosed

Once you have a diagnosis of PCOS, your doctor will most likely continue testing. Periodically checking your blood pressure, cholesterol, glucose, and triglyceride levels can help keep PCOS symptoms in check. Doctors might also recommend routine screenings for depression and anxiety, which can be harmful side effects of dealing with PCOS. There are also other ways you can be active in your management of PCOS after diagnosis without depending on your healthcare provider.

Educate Yourself

You trusted your instincts and advocated for yourself to get the diagnosis, and that shows incredible strength! It can be very hard for women to be outspoken with doctors and healthcare providers, so you are already on the right track by getting your diagnosis.

Keep educating yourself. Your symptoms may change or progress over time, so you want to stay on top of research in the field. This does not mean you have to become a medical expert yourself, but it is helpful to follow the news relating to PCOS to see if any new developments can help you personally. New treatments and research are coming out all of the time, and you do not want to miss anything because you get your diagnosis and think that is the end of it all.

Your diagnosis told you what you are dealing with, but your symptoms are unique to you. Look into the symptoms you have experienced and see how you can better manage them. We will get into that a lot in this book, so you will get a basic foundation of research and learn how you can continue on from this knowledge.

Even if you want to handle your symptoms naturally, without medical intervention, you still want to be aware of what is going on in the medical field relating to

PCOS. This knowledge will empower you on future doctor's visits, so if a method is recommended to you, you might already have some background information about what it will entail.

There is a fear in the unknown, so the more you learn about PCOS at large and your specific symptoms, the stronger you will feel. You will be better prepared to handle your condition, and you will be able to disseminate each individual symptom to its root cause and heal from there.

Assemble a Top-Notch Team

You do not have to suffer through your PCOS journey alone! Assembling a top-notch team can help you every step of the way. While you are educating yourself, also research doctors in your area that are equipped to handle your diagnosis. You do not have to rely on one doctor for everything!

An endocrinologist is a specialist who treats glands, hormones, and metabolism. They can help manage PCOS because they will work to understand why your body might be producing an excess of androgen, or why your metabolism is not breaking down food in a way your body can handle without putting on weight.

An OB/GYN is another doctor you want on your team. An OB/GYN specializes in obstetrics, or pregnancy, and gynecology, or general female reproductive health. They can help you maintain reproductive health from a baseline standard, as well as manage your PCOS symptoms in relation to your periods. OB/GYNs can also help you down the line, when you are trying to conceive.

In larger cities, especially those with research hospitals or medical colleges, you might be able to find both an endocrinologist and an OB/GYN at the same practice. This will be helpful because the specialists can communicate with each other and work together directly as a team to help manage your PCOS. If you cannot find those two specialists in the same practice, make sure you are able to have some open lines of communication between your doctors, whether they share your records or give you information you can share at your next appointment.

Make sure your team consists of doctors you trust and feel comfortable with. PCOS is not your fault, and no doctor should blame you for having the disorder, or shame you for your lifestyle. You should feel confident speaking up and advocating for yourself to members of your team, and you should be able to tell that they are listening to you and taking what you say into consideration. If you want to manage your symptoms naturally, and you have a doctor who is pushing medical intervention, do not be afraid to stop seeing that doctor in favor of finding one who better suits your needs.

After you have your team assembled, make sure you consult them before trying anything on your own. They should know that you plan to change your diet or take on a new exercise regimen before you do so. It is especially crucial to get their input before taking any supplements or medicines! These specialists know you and your body and can advise you what steps will best ease your symptoms. Since you have taken time to research a solid support team, you will trust that these doctors have your best interest in mind when they advise you to do or not do certain things.

Get Support

Once you are diagnosed with PCOS, you will need all kinds of support. You will want to educate your family and friends so they can try to understand what you are going through. Even if you tell them that you have been diagnosed and explain the disorder to them, they might still not know how it affects you. Do not be afraid to tell them about the pain you experience and how it affects you mentally, emotionally, and physically. The more your loved ones know about how PCOS makes you feel, the more they will be able to help you. They might give you grace when it comes to turning down invitations to social engagements, or they might change their own diet to make it easier for you to stick to yours. Never underestimate the support you can get from those close to you, and how it will help you stay on track with your lifestyle changes.

Support from the PCOS community will also be a major help as you navigate your life post-diagnosis. Finding women who are also going through the same things can help you feel understood, while also enabling you to learn more about the condition and the different ways it can affect people. You will be able to share your thoughts, concerns, and progress with a group of like-minded people who can give you tips or just cheer you on. There are many message boards, mailing lists, and social media groups you can join to get this type of support.

Do not feel limited to online communities—seek out support groups in person, too. Your doctor, gynecologist, or other specialists might know of some groups in your city where you can meet other women with PCOS in person. If there is not one, consider starting one! It can be informal, just a monthly meeting at a community center, library, or, after a core group is formed, at people's houses. You can post flyers in doctors' offices or out in your community, or ask your specialists to pass on your email address or phone number to their other PCOS patients. If you want a supportive community and cannot find one, start building it yourself! You might be surprised at how many women around you needed this group until you took the initiative to start it.

Observe Your Body

You might have been observing your body ever since you noticed your initial symptoms, but if you were not doing it before, you definitely want to start post-diagnosis. A lot of women like to keep a diary of things relating to PCOS for easy reference. You can keep a daily food journal, and track how your body feels or how your symptoms may ebb and flow. You might also want to keep track of your menstrual cycle in the same book. Keeping track of these things in one place will help you notice patterns. You might notice that you have more severe symptoms after eating certain foods, or on certain days of your cycle where hormones are higher.

You do not have to write down things about your body to observe it, though. Just be in tune with how you feel throughout the days and weeks. When you feel tired, get some rest, even if you are not usually the type to take a nap. When you feel like you need to get some fresh air, satisfy that urge! Take time to understand your body and be mindful about what it needs. While listening to your body might not solve your problems, understanding it will definitely help you figure out how you can alleviate your PCOS symptoms.

Be Kind to Yourself

Just as it is important that your doctor not blame and shame you for having PCOS, you need to be kind to yourself as well! It is easy to beat yourself up when you are feeling bad, and keep yourself in a dark hole, but that will not make anything better. PCOS can be painful, but letting it take over your mind and emotions is detrimental to your mental health.

There is absolutely nothing to be gained from blaming and shaming yourself for your struggles. In fact, treating yourself unkindly and engaging in negative self-talk could only worsen your condition or at the very least, worsen your emotional state as you manage it. So, when you catch yourself getting low and getting down on yourself, stop. Take a breath. Recognize that negativity will get you nowhere. Remind yourself that patience and optimism are useful to you.

Cut yourself some slack, especially immediately after your diagnosis while you learn the ropes of living with this condition. If you get a goal to exercise five times a week and do not reach that goal every week, do not scold yourself about it. Accept that you are doing the best you can, and vow to improve with time. The same thing goes for your diet—if you eat an unhealthy meal or find yourself snacking one day when you are feeling blue, do not shame yourself for these choices. Acknowledge that you chose poorly and move on, because you can do better with your next meal.

A lot of women with PCOS find that being kind to themselves means making a plan. When you are feeling strong, sit down and map out what makes you feel good. This can be anything from exercise, to eating healthy, to reading in a bubble bath! Nutrition, self-care, or splurging can all be on the list of things you would like to make time for. You can schedule your days to a certain extent, and if you are having a tough time, pick something from the list that makes you feel good. Some days, having a general idea of what you need to do can really help you get out of bed and move. The schedule will give you something to focus on besides your PCOS pain, and since you created it when you were feeling strong, you will know this schedule represents the best you that you can be. It will remind you of what you are capable of, so when you are struggling, it can be a reminder of all that is possible.

Having a specific plan that includes exercise might make you feel more inclined to hit those goals, instead of just shrugging it off and saying you will get to it tomorrow. Meal planning can also be helpful—if you make healthy meals in bigger batches, you will not have to worry about grabbing an unhealthy lunch when you are at work. Having meals prepped ahead of time can also help you stay on a healthy track when you are feeling depressed or anxious due to other symptoms. Even if you are in a bad place mentally, you do not want to throw off your progress by eating junk or drinking alcohol or making other bad choices that will further exacerbate your symptoms. It might feel good to splurge in the moment, but when you are feeling even worse, you will regret those brief moments of excess.

Questions to Ask Your Doctor

Once you are diagnosed with PCOS, your doctor will most likely give you a general background about the condition. You might even get some pamphlets, or resources to use when following up on your own. But before your doctor sends you off with the diagnosis, think of some questions you would like to have answered in person. The internet can be a great way to find information as long as you vet your sources, but sometimes it is best to ask your doctor directly. They know you and your medical history and can give you more specific answers than the internet.

Do I Need to Take Birth Control Pills?

Birth control pills help regulate your menstrual cycle and ovulation by balancing your hormones. The pills can make your period more regular, and also help to alleviate PCOS symptoms like acne and hirsutism. Just because birth control pills can possibly help manage your symptoms does not mean they work for everyone, and it does not mean you have to take them. Some women do not want to take birth control pills for religious or cultural reasons. Some women do not want the risk of side effects, like mood swings, headaches, weight gain or long-term infertility.

If you do not want to take birth control pills, you can still balance your hormones in more natural ways. There are also other medications that can help the body process insulin, which will help promote ovulation while keeping your other symptoms in check. Share any concerns with your doctor and strongly consider their input, since they know your medical history and can help you decide what will work best for you.

How Can I Lower Risk of Complications?

If left untreated, PCOS can lead to increased risks of heart disease, diabetes, and even endometrial cancer. A lesser-known complication of PCOS is sleep apnea, which is associated with extra weight and high levels of androgen. To decrease the possibilities of these conditions, you can follow a treatment plan that you and your doctors develop together. This plan will include lifestyle changes, such as adding in daily exercise, changing your diet, eating nutrient-rich fruits and vegetables, and losing weight.

Losing weight is a major factor in managing your PCOS symptoms because it helps manage your androgen levels and reduce your insulin levels. Insulin resistance is thought to be a cause of PCOS, causes some women to gain weight, and ironically can make it difficult to lose weight. This is why it takes work and strict adherence to your diet and lifestyle to be able to make progress with weight loss.

How Will PCOS Affect My Fertility?

PCOS affects the fertility of over eighty percent of women diagnosed with the condition. If you are thinking of trying to conceive in the future, tell your doctor as soon as possible so you can start making natural changes to your lifestyle to improve your chances of becoming pregnant. Eating a diet with a moderate amount of unprocessed carbohydrates that is rich in antioxidants can help manage PCOS when you are trying to conceive.

Other lifestyle changes like increased physical activity and taking vitamin D supplements can also improve your fertility. It is worth trying these first, with your doctor's approval. If that is not enough to help you get pregnant, you can follow up with your doctor for more information about medication or other medical procedures. There are also assisted reproductive technologies available. Make sure you keep your doctor up to date about what you are doing to get pregnant so that, if the time comes, they can help you with medical intervention.

Just know that most women diagnosed with PCOS and suffering from infertility issues end up getting pregnant and having healthy babies. Instead of worrying about what is to come when you are trying to get pregnant, try to practice self-care so you can be relaxed and stress-free to keep your PCOS symptoms under control.

Chapter 2:

All About PCOS

Polycystic ovarian syndrome, also called PCOS, a hormonal condition that one out of ten women can develop during their childbearing years. PCOS affects a woman's period because the egg might not fully develop or be released as it should. It is the leading cause of female infertility, and also has a variety of other symptoms that affect the body, negatively impacting a woman's physical and mental health.

What is PCOS?

PCOS is a condition that can affect women as early as their first periods and up to perimenopause. Because of the imbalance in hormone levels, PCOS can cause a woman to suffer from infertility, as well as other symptoms that change her body. A higher level of male hormones like androgen and testosterone throws off the normal rhythms of a woman's body, like her menstrual cycle, hair growth, and more.

Three main features of PCOS are cysts in or on the ovaries, irregular or missed periods, and high levels of male hormones. The common thread is the male hormones, which mess up a woman's natural cycle and can cause cysts to grow, though not every woman will develop cysts.

There is no cure for PCOS, but it is possible to manage the symptoms so they do not completely disrupt your lifestyle. It is actually important to keep your symptoms manageable so the condition does not develop into more severe health problems, like diabetes, heart disease, sleep apnea, depression, or cancer.

'Polycystic' means many cysts, but not all women will develop cysts in or on their ovaries. The prevalence of cysts does not affect the severity of symptoms a woman will experience. Many researchers have actually lobbied for the name of the disorder to be changed, because having 'cysts' in the name makes some women, and even doctors, think that PCOS is not an option if no cysts are present.

Cysts can form anywhere in the body, which is why PCOS specifies that they are ovarian cysts. They can also be called follicles, and are fluid-filled sacs that grow on the ovaries. In a healthy woman, they are called 'functional' follicular cysts because the sacs include a mature egg to be released for ovulation. They go away on their own in one to three months. Corpus luteum cysts also usually go away on their own, but are different from follicular cysts. They start with a mature egg to release, but instead of going away after ovulation, when the egg is released, these cysts fill with fluid. They can grow and become painful, even rupturing or twisting the ovary. If you have PCOS and end up taking fertility medication to get pregnant, you will have an increased likelihood of developing these cysts.

In women with PCOS, the follicles contain immature eggs that are not ready to trigger ovulation and be released. The high levels of male hormones often prevent the egg from being released, due to irregular or missed menstrual cycles.

The lack of ovulation disrupts other natural cycles, as well as alters levels of female hormones like estrogen, progesterone, follicle-stimulating hormone, and luteinizing hormone. The ovarian cysts cause the symptoms that make PCOS tough to live with, and can also cause pelvic pain, nausea, high blood pressure, and lower back pain.

Ovarian cysts by themselves are fairly common, and are different from cysts that occur in conjunction with PCOS. Cysts can develop naturally throughout the menstrual cycle, usually during ovulation, and disappear on their own after a few months. Most ovarian cysts are harmless and do not cause any pain or discomfort. A gynecologist can take an ultrasound to see the size and coverage of cysts on the ovaries. They will ask you if you have experienced other symptoms common to PCOS, and then determine the treatment necessary. Most cysts will go away naturally, but if they are cancerous, your doctor will recommend surgery. Taking birth control pills can help prevent new cysts from growing (*Ovarian Cysts*, n.d.).

Symptoms of PCOS

Women with PCOS, before diagnosis, might think that irregular periods, oily skin, feeling tired a lot of the time, and having trouble managing their weight is just a part of normal life. These symptoms can be the result of many health conditions, and not all women suffer the same symptoms. This can make it hard to diagnose PCOS, because most women experience completely different symptoms from each other.

Many women experience irregular periods from the onset of puberty, and do not find out that their cycles should be different until years later. Some women do not realize they have PCOS until they are trying to get pregnant and are having trouble. Symptoms of PCOS vary from woman to woman, so it might take time for individuals to realize what they are dealing with. The symptoms of PCOS are similar to those of many other disorders, so it can be hard to pinpoint the diagnosis.

There is no single test that can diagnose PCOS, so monitoring your symptoms is the best way to learn if you have the condition. When you go to the doctor, they will ask about your symptoms and medical history, so having the information ready will help them determine your diagnosis and help develop a treatment plan.

Triad of Symptoms

There is a triad of symptoms that can help you become aware of your body. Having any number of these symptoms does not mean that you have PCOS, but they are the most common that occur with the condition.

Hirsutism

Hirsutism is the excessive body hair caused by elevated levels of the male hormone androgen. You can check yourself for this symptom by noticing if your body hair is darker or coarser than normal. The hormones might also cause your peach fuzz, the light hair usually found on a woman's face, to be dark and thick like a man's facial hair. You might also find excessive hair growing on your toes, chest, back, and neck.

Anovulation

Anovulation is when your body fails to release an egg during your menstrual cycle. Ovulation usually occurs between days eleven to fourteen of a monthly cycle, but women living with PCOS often do not have a regular cycle, so it can be hard to track the days. When your body fails to release an egg, your cycle and hormones are thrown off track even more. Like hirsutism, this problem can be traced back to high levels of androgen causing an imbalance in a woman's hormones.

If you are having regular monthly cycles, you most likely do not need to worry that you are not ovulating. If you take your concerns about PCOS symptoms to your doctor, they will be able to verify if you are ovulating or not by conducting blood work or a transvaginal ultrasound.

Birth control can be prescribed to regulate your periods and coerce your body to stick to a monthly cycle, but if you are trying to conceive or do not want to be on birth control for other reasons, you do not have to worry about regulating your period. Some drugs used to treat diabetes can help you with insulin resistance, which will also help your body regulate your cycle.

If you are trying to get pregnant, your doctor can prescribe medications that will stimulate ovulation. These will help regulate your cycles while also making your ovaries more viable to release eggs and enable you to carry a pregnancy to term.

Obesity

Obesity is a common symptom of PCOS because the hormonal imbalance and insulin resistance make it hard for you to lose weight. It is hard to know for sure if PCOS causes weight gain, or if being overweight causes PCOS, but it is a symptom that is prevalent in many women regardless of other things they might be experiencing. Even healthy, active women can be diagnosed with PCOS, so weight alone is not enough to determine a diagnosis.

Keeping a healthy lifestyle can be beneficial in managing PCOS symptoms post-diagnosis. Eating a balanced diet can also help keep insulin levels in check, which in turn will help even out hormones while you lose weight. Studies show that even losing ten percent of your body weight can help decrease the severity of symptoms (*Why Irregular Periods, Body Hair, and Obesity Are Common with PCOS*, n.d.).

Symptoms for Diagnosis

Other than these three symptoms you should be aware of, doctors will move forward with diagnosing PCOS if you have two out of three of the following 'official' symptoms:

Irregular Periods

Irregular can mean infrequent or heavier than normal periods that result in a lack of ovulation. Having irregular periods might be painful or it might not, but since your body is not releasing an egg every month, you will most likely have fertility issues.

High Levels of Androgens

All women have some androgens, or male hormones, in their blood, but women with PCOS have higher levels than normal. These androgens cause excessive body hair growth, especially on the face. The hormones can also cause hair loss.

Ovarian Cysts

Having cysts, or follicles, on the ovaries, is normal for most women. Cysts can develop during ovulation and go away on their own in time. However, if you have more than twelve on your ovaries, it could be a sign of PCOS. Doctors will check for cysts by conducting an ultrasound. Not all women with PCOS have cysts, which is why only two out of three of these symptoms need to be met for diagnosis.

Causes of PCOS

No one can pinpoint exactly what causes PCOS, but research has shown a few factors are most common in women diagnosed with PCOS. Since the male hormone levels are much higher than other hormones in women who have PCOS, the most common thought is that the hormones throw off the whole body's balance to cause PCOS. But are the hormones increased because of how the woman lives or what she eats, or is it genetic? Research shows that PCOS runs in families, so there is a strong reason to believe that it is a genetic condition.

Almost seventy percent of women who have PCOS also have insulin resistance. Insulin is needed to break down sugars from food into energy the body can use up. If your body cannot convert insulin into energy, the body stores the sugars while demanding more insulin. This usually presents in the form of cravings, most likely for sweets and other unhealthy foods. The pancreas produces more insulin to try and compensate. This excess insulin triggers the body to produce more androgen, which in turn sets off other PCOS symptoms like irregular periods, hirsutism, and a lack of ovulation.

It is hard to tell if obesity is a cause of or result of PCOS. Insulin resistance makes it harder for women to lose weight, but a lot of women who are diagnosed with PCOS are overweight. So were they overweight and then began to suffer from PCOS, or did undiagnosed PCOS cause women to gain weight and be unable to easily lose it? Being overweight also makes a woman more likely to suffer from inflammation. Studies have found that inflammation can raise the levels of androgen in the body, which will then set off the other triggers of PCOS.

While it is difficult to find just one cause of PCOS, the way that all of the potential causes work together tends to show that the condition is just a perfect storm of things going awry compared to the body's usual balance of hormones, weight, and insulin processing. If your mother or sister has PCOS, you are likely to have it as well. Prenatal exposure to androgen and testosterone may prime your body to produce high levels of these hormones. There are even studies that show stress and environmental factors like diet, exercise, and pollution you may breathe play a role in the development of PCOS.

Treatments for PCOS

PCOS treatment depends on many different things, such as your age, your symptoms, and if you think you will try to get pregnant in the near future. Treatment can be individualized for each symptom you experience, like irregular periods, body hair, acne, and insulin levels. There are also fertility treatments that can help you get pregnant.

Whether you want to try medication or other treatments prescribed by your doctor, or things you can do more naturally on your own, you will need to talk to your specialist and make sure you find the right treatment for you. Be honest about your goals for treatment—are you trying to get rid of unwanted hair or acne, or are you trying to get pregnant? Your goal will determine what treatment is best for you.

Prescribed Treatments

Your doctor might offer some medical options to manage your PCOS symptoms. Your doctor or specialist best knows your medical history and your body, so they will prescribe medications that will best be able to help in your situation.

Hormonal Birth Control

Treatment of PCOS focuses on regulating your menstrual cycle, because this will help keep your hormones in balance, and will increase your chances at ovulation and getting pregnant naturally. Hormonal birth control is the standard way that doctors help women regulate their cycles, though of course this is a counter-intuitive treatment if you plan to get pregnant soon!

Hormonal birth control relies on you taking a pill at the same time every day to work as effective birth control, because they prevent you from ovulating. These pills contain hormones, typically estrogen and progestin, that help regulate your body to follow a twenty-one day cycle, then a week of non-hormonal pills for your period. There are also extended-cycle pills that allow you to take pills with hormones for twelve weeks, then take pills without hormones for one week to allow you to have a period. This means you will only have menstrual cycles three or four times a year.

Progestin-only pills are also available, but there are no inactive pills in the cycle. This means every pill has the hormone, so you may not get a period with this pill. Since this pill does not contain estrogen, it might not be a good option to help PCOS-sufferers manage their symptoms. Your doctor will know if this type of pill will be effective for you, based on your hormone levels, menstrual history, and if you plan on trying to get pregnant soon.

Certain medications and supplements make birth control less effective. If you are only using it to manage your PCOS symptoms, it might not be as big of a concern, but you will still want to tell your doctor if you are taking anything else. Known supplements that interfere with birth control include antiseizure medications, antibiotics, and St. John's Wort.

In addition to managing your PCOS symptoms, hormonal birth control pills have other benefits. These include protecting you from ectopic pregnancies, non-cancerous breast growths, anemia, menstrual cramps, and endometrial and ovarian cancers. There are side effects of taking birth control pills, and they vary from woman to woman. They can include mood swings, low sex drive, breast tenderness, nausea, and spotting between periods.

There is also an increased risk of blood clots if you are taking the pill, which can lead to heart attacks, pulmonary embolisms, and strokes. These are low risks, and taking the pills with your doctor's supervision will help you stay on top of any potential side effects you may feel. If you start to feel strange or sick while taking the pill, tell your doctor so you can try a different type of pill, or work to manage your symptoms in another way.

Hormonal birth control is not limited to pills. There are hormonal birth control patches that you wear on your skin for twenty-one days, then remove to have a regular menstrual cycle. Like the pill, these patches contain estrogen and progestin, and help level out your hormones and promote a regulated cycle.

Vaginal rings are another option of hormonal birth control. You insert it into your vagina and leave it for twenty-one days, then take it out for seven days to have a period. When your period ends, you will insert a new ring to get the hormonal benefits again.

If you do not want to take an oral contraceptive, ask your doctor if other hormonal options, like a patch or ring, are options for you. Some IUDs (intrauterine devices) might also be effective, though they only contain progestin, so are more like progestin-only pills than combination pills that include estrogen.

Progestin Therapy

Progestin can still be an option to manage your PCOS symptoms even if you do not opt for birth control. You can take this hormone daily for ten or fourteen days every month or two to regulate your periods and even protect against endometrial cancer. Progestin promotes a thickening in the lining of your uterus. If the hormone is discontinued, then the uterus sloughs off the lining, causing your period to start. It has been effective in stimulating the bleeding that signals the beginning of your menstrual cycle.

Progestin does not balance out your androgen hormones, so it might not help ease any symptoms that result from having higher male hormone levels. Progestin on its own does not prevent pregnancy, so if you are trying to conceive or do not want to take birth control pills for that reason, progestin therapy might be a good alternative for you.

However, a study has shown that progestin therapy may have reduced pregnancy chances. Women who did not do a cycle of progestin therapy before starting fertility drugs were four times more likely to get pregnant than women who had progestin therapy (*Progestin treatment for polycystic ovarian syndrome may reduce pregnancy chances*, 2015). So while progestin on its own will not effectively prevent pregnancy as a birth control pill would, you might not want to take a chance with progestin therapy. Be sure to discuss any concerns with your doctor, who might have more data about such studies.

Anti-Androgen Medications

Spironolactone is an anti-androgen medication commonly used to manage PCOS symptoms, though the medicine is not specifically made for that purpose. Since it decreases the levels of androgen in your body, it curbs some of the symptoms related to the male hormone, especially hirsutism, or excess hair. It takes about six months for the difference to be noticeable, but the hair starts growing back in finer and lighter. Spironolactone also helps eliminate your acne, and those results are typically seen more quickly than any change in hirsutism.

This medication is usually prescribed along with birth control pills because it is not safe to take during pregnancy. If you are not taking birth control pills, be sure you are using a different effective method of birth control while taking spironolactone.

Metformin

Metformin is a medication used to treat type 2 diabetes. It makes the body more sensitive to insulin by lowering insulin, glucose, and androgen levels while improving insulin resistance. The Food and Drug Administration has not authorized the use of metformin for PCOS, but since insulin resistance is a symptom of PCOS, it makes sense that the medication can help manage that symptom. Some women who have tried metformin found that it restarted their periods and promoted ovulation, and also helped them lose weight.

Other medications that support ovulation include:
- clomiphene, which modulates estrogen levels
- letrozole, which stimulates the ovaries

- gonadotropins, which are hormones that stimulate the follicles.

Natural Treatments

In addition to the medical options given above, there are ways you can try to manage your PCOS symptoms on your own, at home, with little or no extra supplies needed.

Weight Loss

The most common treatment that is usually the first thing suggested is to lose weight. Even if you are not obese, losing five to ten percent of your body weight can help you manage other symptoms. Losing this weight can even help you ovulate regularly, if that has been an issue you are struggling with. Losing weight will also help your medications work more efficiently, if you choose to treat any of your conditions with medicine.

Losing weight is hard enough, but if you are dealing with the hormone levels and insulin resistance associated with PCOS, you might struggle even more to lose weight and keep it off. The most important thing is to stay on track with healthy eating habits and regular exercise. It is easy to feel like you are doing a lot of work for no payout, but regular work will make your body healthier to handle the symptoms, and in time you will be able to actually see the difference. Working hard to lose weight and keep it off will also help your body be healthier to fight back against more severe disorders you are susceptible to, just because you have PCOS. These conditions include diabetes, heart disease, high cholesterol, and strokes.

Hair Removal

You can remove hair on your own by trying hair removal creams or other over the counter products. Depilatories are creams or gels that break down the protein of hair so it falls out of your skin. If you are unhappy with options at drugstores or beauty supply stores, you can ask your doctor to prescribe eflornithine HCl cream, which is a skin treatment that slows down hair growth when you apply it to places where unwanted hair is growing. You can also look into laser hair removal, which destroys the hair follicles, or electrolysis, which removes hairs at their roots. Keep in mind these must be done by professionals and might not be covered by insurance. Sometimes birth control or other hormonal medications might lower your androgen levels and, in turn, diminish the darkness or thickness of your hair growth.

Supplements

Some women have noticed positive changes in the severity of PCOS symptoms after taking natural supplements. Supplements can help balance hormones and regulate your body, but you should check with your doctor before taking any. They might interfere with other medications you are on, or they might not be a good choice for your medical situation.

Cinnamon extract has been shown to improve your body's insulin resistance and can even help with fertility. Turmeric is another supplement that can naturally have positive effects on insulin resistance, and also has anti-inflammatory qualities. Zinc can boost your fertility as well as your immune system, and even helps balance out both excess hair growth and hair loss. You can get more zinc by adding seafood, beans, red meat, and tree nuts to your diet.

Many women with PCOS have low levels of vitamin D, so taking a supplement might help balance your system. Calcium can also help regulate your period and promote ovulation.

Adaptogen Herbs

Adaptogen herbs help your body balance androgen levels naturally and promote a regular menstrual cycle. Maca root is an herb traditionally used to boost fertility and libido. When taken by a woman with PCOS, maca root can lower cortisol levels and balance androgens. Ashwagandha is an herb similar to maca root, and it also has anti-depressive characteristics that can be useful in terms of self-care with PCOS.

Holy basil can help prevent weight gain and lower your blood sugar. Licorice root is an anti-inflammatory that balances hormones and metabolizes sugar, which can be a positive benefit for people with insulin resistance. Tribulus terrestris is a supplement that stimulates ovulation; it can even decrease the number of ovarian cysts.

Probiotics

Probiotics are a popular, natural way to improve gut health, and this can benefit women diagnosed with PCOS. Insulin resistance and androgen levels can affect the healthy bacteria in your stomach, so women with PCOS might have trouble with digestion (Shamasbi et al., 2019).

Probiotics also reduce inflammation and regulate androgen and estrogen levels. Foods with high probiotic content include garlic, asparagus, bananas, onions, kimchi, artichokes, and kombucha. You can also take probiotic supplements in pill form or as yogurt drinks.

Possible Complications of PCOS Symptoms

Having PCOS cannot only have painful symptoms you live with every day, but it also increases your risks of other, more serious complications. Researchers still are not sure if PCOS causes these complications, if these complications cause PCOS, or if there are other, possibly underlying and undiagnosed issues, that cause PCOS and other health problems. As you read through these complications, you will notice that some of the conditions have symptoms in common with PCOS. This can be a good thing, because some of the ways you can manage PCOS symptoms will also help you keep these problems in check. However, it does make it clear that there is a vicious cycle linking PCOS and other hormonal problems together.

Infertility

Having PCOS may make it difficult to get pregnant, but it does not make you completely infertile. Since hormone levels associated with PCOS disrupt your cycle and might hinder ovulation, it might take you longer to get pregnant. If you have cysts in or on your ovaries, they might prevent regular ovulation, when your ovaries release an egg in the middle of your menstrual cycle to be fertilized. If you do not release a healthy egg to be fertilized by sperm, you will not be able to get pregnant easily.

If you have been trying to conceive over many cycles, your PCOS might be affecting your ability to get pregnant. Your doctor might recommend a lifestyle change or some fertility treatments, such as oral medications like clomiphene or letrozole, or injections like gonadotropins. Fertility injections push the body to release more than one egg a month, so the chances of getting pregnant are increased. If none of these treatments work, there are assisted reproductive technologies that can help you have a baby.

Bloating

Women who have PCOS can also suffer from bloating, though often this is triggered by certain foods. The carbohydrate raffinose is hard for people with PCOS to digest, so it causes gas and bloating. Foods with raffinose include Brussels sprouts, broccoli, cauliflower, cabbage, beans, and asparagus. If you are lactose intolerant, foods with dairy can cause gas and bloating issues. Some whole-grain foods may also be difficult to digest, along with carbonated drinks, fruits high in sugar, and other artificially sweetened foods. Keeping a food diary might help you notice what foods trigger both PCOS symptoms and bloating, so you can take them out of your diet for fewer complications.

Uterine Bleeding

PCOS can cause your periods to be heavier than they normally would and last longer than normal, typically at least seven days, if not more. This type of heavy period is called menorrhagia, and it is usually caused by low levels of progesterone.

Uterine bleeding can also be caused by a lack of ovulation. When the endometrium, the lining of the uterus, gets thicker, it builds up because of estrogen production. Typically, progesterone would be released from the ovary after ovulation, but with PCOS causing a hormonal imbalance and preventing ovulation, the uterus keeps its thick lining. Taking oral contraceptives can help slough this thick lining away and prevent the irregular bleeding.

Diabetes

More than half of all women diagnosed with PCOS will develop prediabetes or diabetes before they turn forty. PCOS causes insulin resistance, and that creates a negative reaction in the endocrine system that can sometimes lead to type 2 diabetes. Type 2 diabetes typically occurs if the body is resistant to insulin or if too much insulin is being produced, both of which are options for people diagnosed with PCOS.

Women with PCOS are four to eight times more likely to become diabetic over time, but since doctors are aware, they will periodically screen you to make sure your insulin levels are okay. Diabetes is preventable with exercise and a healthy diet, which are also good ways to manage PCOS symptoms. Birth control pills and metformin can also help both PCOS symptoms and hormone levels related to diabetes. It is not guaranteed that one treatment can alleviate both PCOS and diabetes conditions, but there is definitely some overlap in what might help.

Pregnant women with PCOS are more likely to get gestational diabetes. This is when you are first diagnosed with diabetes during pregnancy, and causes high blood sugar that can affect both your health and your baby's. You can control your blood sugar by eating healthy foods and exercising. If that does not get your glucose levels under control, your doctor may prescribe medication that is safe to take while pregnant. After delivering your baby, your glucose levels may go back to normal. Once you have had gestational diabetes, your doctor will schedule regular screenings to make sure you do not develop type 2 diabetes later.

High Blood Pressure

High blood pressure is also called hypertension, and is a serious risk to women with PCOS. There are not many warning signs for hypertension, so you will want to make sure any of your new doctors and specialists are aware of your PCOS diagnosis and can keep an eye on your blood pressure. Doctors typically take your blood pressure at the beginning of any appointment, and will be aware if your numbers are higher than they should be considering your medical history.

High blood pressure can cause damage to your blood vessels and other organs, cause kidney damage, give you vision problems, or even cause heart attacks and strokes. Risks are increased if, in addition to PCOS, you are a smoker, overweight, African-American, older, or have a history of high blood pressure in your family.

You can help keep your blood pressure low by exercising, abstaining from alcohol, and eating healthy foods. Foods to avoid include anything with high salt content, while you should eat more fruits and vegetables. Fruits and vegetables have nutrients like magnesium, potassium, and calcium, which can be taken as supplements, but are more beneficial if you get them directly from the source. Seeds, nuts, and legumes are also good choices to add to your diet because they are good sources of fiber.

If you add these foods to your diet, increase your physical activity, and still suffer from high blood pressure, talk to your doctor about medications that may be able to help you. Diuretics help eliminate excess salt and water from your body, which will lower your blood pressure. Spironolactone is an example of a diuretic, and is also used to treat PCOS for its anti-androgen properties.

Calcium channel blockers work to lower blood pressure by preventing calcium buildup in your blood vessels. When there is calcium blocking your blood vessels, your heart has to pump that much harder to get blood to flow through your body, and that raises your blood pressure. Beta blockers are also effective medications to lower your blood pressure by blocking epinephrine, or adrenaline, to slow your heartbeat. ACE inhibitors expand your blood vessels so your blood can flow easily through your body instead of struggling to push through, which increases your blood pressure.

High Cholesterol

There are good cholesterols, high-density lipoproteins (HDL), and bad cholesterols, or low-density lipoproteins (LDL). High cholesterol is harmful if you have low levels of HDL and high levels of LDL. It might seem confusing, but an easy way to keep things straight is to remember that you should have high levels of high-density lipoproteins, because they actually can clear the build-up of LDL from your blood vessels. If you have low levels of HDL, you have fewer lipoproteins that can clear your arteries and prevent heart attacks and strokes.

Then it is only logical that high levels of LDL just mean that there are more bad lipoproteins causing that buildup in your arteries. But how can you know what your lipid levels are, and how can you prevent LDL build up in your arteries?

Over seventy percent of women diagnosed with PCOS are at risk for high cholesterol and abnormal triglyceride levels. The American Heart Association recommends that people over twenty years of age get their lipid levels checked every four years, but if you have PCOS then your doctor will probably perform these tests more often.

Your cholesterol and lipid levels may be higher because of your weight, your insulin resistance, or your hormone levels. We know that this triad of symptoms is a hallmark of PCOS, so it makes sense that they could also cause you to have high cholesterol.

Managing your cholesterol levels can be done in the same way you are managing many of your other PCOS symptoms: with a healthy diet, plenty of exercise, and losing weight. Your cholesterol levels can also be managed by keeping your stress under control and giving up cigarettes if you are a smoker.

If you make these lifestyle changes but your cholesterol levels do not improve, your doctor may prescribe medication to help you manage this problem. Statins, bile acid resins, fibric acids, and absorption inhibitors are a few examples of these medicines. As of now, no research has shown that these pills help manage any PCOS symptoms other than keeping your cholesterol in check. Some of the medicines cannot be taken in conjunction with other vitamins or medications, so make sure your doctor knows all of the medicines and supplements you are taking to manage other symptoms.

Sleep Apnea

Sleep apnea is a disorder where you stop breathing for brief periods in your sleep. It messes up your body's oxygen flow and disrupts your sleep cycle. Higher levels of male hormones like testosterone have led to sleep disturbances like sleep apnea. Being overweight can also increase the likelihood that you will experience sleep apnea. And of course, both male hormones and weight struggles are common symptoms of PCOS.

Because it messes up your body's oxygen supply, sleep apnea can cause further complications, like high blood pressure, lower pain tolerance, heart disease, weight problems, and mood swings.

Before you experience any of these complications, you might notice some symptoms of sleep apnea. These include feeling very tired during the daytime and having trouble focusing. People who live with you might notice that you are snoring when you are asleep—not regular snoring, but loud, uneven, disruptive snoring. Someone who sleeps with you might also notice if there are periods where you stop breathing while you are asleep.

If you are having any of these symptoms, either that you notice or that your partner notices, inform your doctor so you can participate in a sleep study. Researchers conducting the study will monitor your breathing, heartbeat, and brain activity for any abnormalities. If you do have sleep apnea, there are breathing treatments you can use while you sleep, like a CPAP machine, that will keep your breathing steady.

Continuous positive airway pressure (CPAP) machines include a mask or nose piece that you wear when you sleep. A hose connects your mask to the machine to provide constant air to you while you sleep. The machine pushes the air through the hose at a specific pressure that keeps your airways open. This will prevent you from snoring or stopping breathing while you sleep. The CPAP machine might sound cumbersome, but you will get used to it in time. If you find that the CPAP machine is not working for you, ask your doctor about other options. You can try alternatives like other oral appliances, nasal valve therapy, bilevel positive airway pressure (BiPAP), or even surgery.

Depression and Anxiety

Symptoms of PCOS can cause you a lot of physical pain, and it only makes sense that this physical pain also negatively impacts your emotional and mental well-being. In fact, women diagnosed with PCOS are three to five times more likely to experience depression and anxiety than other women, and it is usually more severe. Doctors are not sure of a specific reason behind this statistic, but it is something you should be aware of as you manage other symptoms. You might already be familiar with these feelings, possibly even battling them while you suffered the pain without knowing your diagnosis.

Some doctors think that PCOS can cause depression and anxiety due to the hormonal imbalance it makes in your body. It is also possible that just the fact that you are living with an incurable condition is enough to depress you, and cause you to have anxiety about all the detrimental aspects of the disorder and what it might mean for your future.

Having unwanted excess hair, especially if it is hair on your face or other obvious locations, can make you feel anxious and depressed about how others see you, and cause you to suffer from low self-esteem. Struggling with infertility can also make you feel depressed, especially if you feel ready to start your own family and view your infertility as a personal failure.

The hormonal imbalance caused by PCOS can affect your serotonin levels, which impacts your neurotransmitters. Serotonin plays a big part in depression and anxiety, and research has shown that people with PCOS have low serotonin levels.

You can treat your depression and anxiety just as people who do not have PCOS might do. That includes increased levels of activity. Exercising and getting outside for sunlight and fresh air has been shown to make a huge difference in the mental state of people with depression and anxiety. Eating better makes your body feel good, and that will affect your mental health as well.

Making time for self-care and giving yourself the grace to say no to certain commitments or to make certain mistakes can also make a huge difference in your depression and anxiety. If you feel like you always need to go to the party, or if you have a fear of missing out, you might bully yourself into going to events when you really should have stayed home and taken some time to relax. Holding yourself to impossible standards, in your social life, work life, and personal life, is also detrimental to your emotional well-being, so you should make sure you are being kind to yourself and cutting yourself some slack.

If your problems persist, do not be afraid to talk to your doctor. Talk therapy might help you air your problems and get an external point of view about things that have been bothering you. Some people have also found benefits in alternative therapies, like practicing mindfulness or acupuncture. Make sure to do your research and talk to your doctor before you try something new with your body.

You can also take medication to manage your depression and anxiety. Metformin, which improves insulin resistance, has also been shown to be effective in treating depression. This means you can take one medication and get a lot of benefits from it! Otherwise, make sure your psychiatrist or specialist knows about your PCOS diagnosis and any other medications or supplements you are taking before they prescribe anything extra for your depression and anxiety.

While the research on PCOS and mental health focuses on anxiety and depression, women with this diagnosis have also noted suffering from bipolar disorder, obsessive-compulsive disorder (OCD), and eating disorders. Eating disorders are especially common since so many PCOS symptoms can be managed by watching your diet. It might become something obsessive you feel like you need to always think about and struggle to control, and that degree of involvement can be unhealthy mentally and lead to disordered eating. If you feel like any of these problems are weighing heavily on you, speak to your doctor about possible treatments.

Endometrial Cancer

Because having PCOS means you have higher levels of androgen and estrogen compared to levels of progesterone, you are more at risk for developing endometrial cancer. This cancer develops when the cells of the endometrium, or the lining of the uterus, grow abnormally. During a woman's menstrual cycle, hormones cause the endometrium to thicken so that it can nurture an embryo as it grows into a fetus. If an egg is not fertilized, a woman produces less estrogen and more progesterone so the endometrium will thin back out and be shed as a period.

Endometrial cancer starts in the lining inside the uterus, but type 2 endometrial cancer cells, which make up fewer cases, can spread to the outside of the uterus and elsewhere in the body. There are different types of endometrial cancer cells, including:

- Adenocarcinoma
- Uterine carcinosarcoma
- Small cell carcinoma
- Serous carcinoma
- Transitional carcinoma
- Squamous cell carcinoma

Risk factors for endometrial cancer include many of the symptoms of PCOS, such as obesity, diet and exercise, hormone levels, type 2 diabetes, and family history. Because women with PCOS produce a different level of estrogen compared to progesterone, they are at a higher risk for developing endometrial cancer. Pregnancies help decrease the likelihood of developing endometrial cancer, but since women with PCOS have a harder time getting pregnant, this also increases their risk (*Endometrial Cancer*, n.d.).

Endometrial cancer can be detected early if you notice any unusual vaginal bleeding or discharge. Since these are common occurrences with PCOS, it can be tough for a woman to notice anything different than how her cycles usually go. Make sure that any new doctors or specialists are aware that you have PCOS so they can do testing for possible tumors in and on your uterus. It is important to keep in mind that not all tumors will cause discharge or side effects, so you might want to set up a regular testing schedule with your doctor, especially if you have a family history of women with cancer.

If you are experiencing symptoms of endometrial cancer or want to be tested because of your PCOS diagnosis, see your gynecologist or make an appointment for a gynecologic oncologist, who specializes in treatment of female reproductive cancers. The specialist will look over your medical history, request an ultrasound, and take a sample of your endometrium. If the doctor suspects the cancer has spread, they might x-ray other parts of your body.

Treatment for endometrial cancer is similar to other cancers, with surgery, chemotherapy, radiation, immunotherapy, and hormone therapy being options, depending on the severity of the tumors, your age, your overall health, and whether you plan on having children.

Nonalcoholic Steatohepatitis

Nonalcoholic steatohepatitis (NASH) is also called nonalcoholic fatty liver disease (NAFLD), or just fatty liver. Obesity and insulin resistance are considered the two major factors that contribute to fatty liver, so it makes sense that it is a common complication in patients with PCOS. When excess fat is stored in the liver, it causes damage and inflammation. The liver is meant to function as a purification organ, not for storage, so when it keeps fat instead of filtering out toxins, it will cause damage.

Factors contributing to NAFLD include extra weight, high cholesterol levels, an inactive lifestyle, a diet high in fat and sugar, and genetics. You will notice that many of these factors are similar to symptoms of PCOS, so it is understandable that women with PCOS also are more likely to develop NAFLD. High androgen levels have also been linked to fatty liver, and that is another PCOS symptom. Just like managing PCOS symptoms, you can try to prevent fatty liver by eating a healthy diet, losing weight, and being active. You can also take fish oil to prevent NAFLD. You can eat salmon, trout, and tuna, but it is hard to eat enough to really boost your omega-

3 levels, so you might want to take a fish oil supplement.

Metabolic Syndrome

PCOS and metabolic syndrome share many factors, such as insulin resistance, high cholesterol, and obesity, making it a likely complication for women diagnosed with PCOS. Metabolic syndrome is not really one condition, but rather a cluster of many issues that work together to potentially cause cardiovascular problems and other health concerns.

Women with PCOS are over eleven times more likely to develop metabolic syndrome than women without PCOS. Doctors will diagnose you with metabolic syndrome if you display three or more of these characteristics:

- overweight
- high blood glucose levels
- high triglyceride levels
- low HDL cholesterol levels
- high blood pressure

The risk of metabolic syndrome increases with age. By the time women reach menopause, they are at a higher risk for metabolic syndrome due to the increase in testosterone production.

If you are overweight, you are at a higher risk for metabolic syndrome, though you do not have to be overweight to develop the condition. Eating an unhealthy diet, especially if you eat carbohydrates and fried foods. In recent years, researchers have found that metabolic syndrome is more prevalent in adolescents. Since PCOS symptoms also start when females begin their menstrual cycle as adolescents, it is especially important for this population to be aware of the symptoms and possible side effects of metabolic syndrome.

Effects on Pregnancy

Seventy to eighty percent of women with PCOS struggle with infertility, so it seems especially cruel that they are also at high risk for complications with pregnancy. Symptoms of PCOS, like increased androgens and metabolic syndrome, might also cause issues with the newborn that would require them to be closely watched in a neonatal intensive care unit after birth. There are many different effects on pregnancy that PCOS can cause.

To try and reduce your chance of having problems during pregnancy, you can reach a healthy weight before getting pregnant, and maintain a healthy weight gain during pregnancy. You can also keep your blood sugar levels in a healthy range by eating right, exercising, and losing weight. Tell your doctor if you plan on getting pregnant so they can help you reach these goals, even if it means prescribing medicine to help you get on the right track. You can also talk to your doctor about taking folic acid to help increase your chances of ovulation when you are trying to conceive. You can keep taking folic acid throughout your pregnancy to diminish the chances of your baby being born with birth defects.

Miscarriage

It is a gruesome statistic, but anywhere between thirty to fifty percent of women with PCOS will experience first trimester miscarriages. This is compared to a ten to twenty perfect chance of first trimester miscarriages in women without PCOS. Some studies show that metformin may reduce your risk of an early miscarriage. Metformin is also a potential treatment for PCOS symptoms because it increases your body's sensitivity to insulin by lowering insulin, glucose, and androgen levels while improving insulin resistance.

Insulin resistance, high testosterone levels, obesity, and genetic factors contribute to miscarriages, and you will notice that many of these are also symptoms of PCOS. While not guaranteed to reduce your risk of miscarriage, losing weight, exercising, and eating a healthy diet will increase your possibilities of carrying a pregnancy to term. Since these are also ways to manage PCOS symptoms, it will most likely be no problem for you to adhere to.

It is not possible to prevent a miscarriage, because they are often due to a genetic abnormality that would keep the baby from living even if you carried it to term. So it is important to take care of yourself as much as possible to reduce stress and follow your doctor's advice about your health, diet, and if you need to be on bed rest.

Pregnancy-Induced High Blood Pressure

High blood pressure during pregnancy can lead to many different complications. Gestational hypertension is when women have high blood pressure after twenty weeks of pregnancy. There are rarely warning signs for this condition, and it can lead to preeclampsia.

Chronic hypertension is high blood pressure that you might have had before pregnancy, or that shows up before the twenty week mark of pregnancy. Since high blood pressure does not often showcase any symptoms, you might not know you have it, or you might not be able to pinpoint when you developed it.

High blood pressure during pregnancy is a problem because it can lead to decreased blood flow to the placenta. This means your baby will get less oxygen and nutrients, meaning they will grow slowly and be born with a low birth weight. An undeveloped baby can also lead to a premature birth, which might mean your baby will have to be on a breathing machine or cared for extensively in the neonatal intensive care unit.

Your doctor will monitor your blood pressure at your prenatal appointments, and you can also keep track of it yourself at home. Some blood pressure medications are safe to take during pregnancy, but you will want to double-check with your doctor before trying any medication. Staying active and eating right can also help you lower your blood pressure. Know that high blood pressure can lead to preeclampsia and preterm birth, so make sure you research these conditions as well. More detail will be given on both later on in this section.

Gestational Diabetes

Gestational diabetes occurs when you are diagnosed with diabetes for the first time during pregnancy. The high blood sugar that is common in diabetes can affect both your health and your baby's. You can maintain an ideal blood sugar level by eating healthy foods and exercising regularly. If those lifestyle changes do not get your glucose levels under control, you may want to see if your doctor can prescribe medication that is safe to take while pregnant.

Warning signs of gestational diabetes include frequent urination, unquenchable thirst, fatigue, nausea, and various skin, vaginal, or bladder infections. Women who do not make enough insulin or are obese are more prone to develop gestational diabetes. You can also get gestational diabetes if you gain too much weight during pregnancy. Even if you do not have a resistance to insulin before pregnancy, you can develop it because your body uses insulin differently when you are pregnant.

You can watch your diet when you are pregnant to try and prevent gestational diabetes from developing. This means you should cut out any processed food and white bread, eat protein with every meal, eat more fruits and vegetables, and serve manageable portions to prevent overeating.

Having gestational diabetes can be detrimental for both you and your baby. It may cause your baby to gain weight, which will make the delivery more difficult. The baby might get stuck, cause more bleeding, or have trouble managing their own blood sugar after birth.

While you cannot typically get rid of gestational diabetes while pregnant, your glucose levels may go back to normal after you deliver the baby. If you have had gestational diabetes during pregnancy, your doctor will check you and your baby for diabetes, and will schedule regular screenings to make sure you do not develop type 2 diabetes later.

Preeclampsia

Preeclampsia is thought to develop because there are so many new blood vessels forming to send blood to the placenta. When women have preeclampsia, there is usually some developmental problem with the new blood vessels so they do not function properly. They might be narrower than other blood vessels, which can limit how much blood is flowing through the vessels to the placenta.

It is a complication that centers around high blood pressure and liver or kidney damage. Even if you have had healthy blood pressure for the first part of your pregnancy, preeclampsia can develop suddenly at twenty weeks. If untreated, preeclampsia can be fatal for you and your baby. You might have to deliver your baby early to reduce the risks, but even after giving birth it might still take time for you to get healthy. It can be a major problem if you are diagnosed with preeclampsia too early in the pregnancy to give birth. You want your baby to be mature and developed enough to survive on its own, but waiting too long is a risk for both of you.

Risk factors for preeclampsia include a family history of the condition, hypertension, if it is your first pregnancy, or your first pregnancy with a new partner, if you are either very young or over thirty-five, obesity, carrying multiples, or being impregnated by in vitro fertilization. If you are having babies less than two years apart or more than ten years apart then that also might put you at risk for preeclampsia.

Preeclampsia can develop suddenly or slowly, without showing any symptoms either way. If any symptoms present, it is usually as high blood pressure, so it is important to closely monitor your blood pressure throughout your pregnancy. You will want to look out for other symptoms, in case they become prevalent, such as:

- protein in your urine
- kidney problems
- severe headaches
- blurred vision or light sensitivity
- abdominal pain under your ribs
- nausea and vomiting
- less frequent urination
- shortness of breath

Complications of preeclampsia include fetal growth restriction, which can mean your baby is born with a low birth weight because the condition prevented your baby from getting enough blood, oxygen, or nutrients. You might have to have a preterm birth to save both you and the baby, with prematurity causing potential issues for the baby's survival. The baby may have breathing issues or need supplemental nutrients.

Your risk for placental abruption is increased if you have preeclampsia. This is when the placenta separates from the uterus wall before delivery, causing severe bleeding that is life-threatening for both you and your baby. Preeclampsia can also lead to cardiovascular disease and other organ damage, depending on the severity.

Your doctor will monitor your blood pressure at your regular prenatal visits, but if you experience any of the symptoms listed above, call your doctor immediately and go to the emergency room. If you are unsure if some of these symptoms, like nausea, shortness of breath, and other aches are common pregnancy complaints or actually symptoms of preeclampsia, take notes on how you feel and be sure to share the information with your doctor.

Preterm Birth

A baby is considered preterm if they are born before thirty-seven weeks gestation, because a full-term pregnancy is typically forty weeks long. Women with PCOS are more at risk for preterm births because of all the complications PCOS exposes them to. High blood pressure, gestational diabetes, and preeclampsia can all potentially lead to preterm birth.

Preterm birth might mean your baby is born underweight, cannot breathe on its own, or has to stay in the neonatal intensive care unit to be monitored. They may need to get supplements and nutrients through an intravenous tube. If a baby is born too early, it might not be able to survive on its own. Babies who do survive might have long-term disabilities that affect them intellectually, developmentally, or physically.

Cesarean Delivery

A cesarean delivery, or c-section, is when a baby is delivered through surgery instead of through vaginal birth. Because a cesarean delivery is a surgical procedure, it takes longer for the mother to heal from the incision. The surgery cuts through the abdomen and uterus to remove the baby from the womb. The incision is sewn up with stitches that will dissolve naturally as the skin heals. C-sections are fairly common for all women, but happen frequently to women with PCOS because of factors that complicate a natural birth, like the baby's weight, high blood pressure, preeclampsia, and more.

C-sections are commonly done if labor is not progressing naturally or the baby's health is at risk. Cesareans are also done if the woman is giving birth to multiple babies, or if the baby has a high birth weight. If there are any disruptions in the placenta, such as abruption from preeclampsia, a c-section might be necessary to save both the mother's and the baby's lives. They are also done if the mother has an infection, like HIV or herpes, that can be passed to the baby through a vaginal birth.

Fetal Macrosomia

Fetal macrosomia is when a baby is born much larger than the typical newborn. A baby that is larger than eight pounds, thirteen ounces is considered bigger than average, regardless of their age at the time of delivery. Less than ten percent of babies in the world are born weighing more than eight pounds and thirteen ounces. Complications increase for babies that are born weighing over nine pounds, fifteen ounces.

Vaginal delivery is complicated if the baby is born with fetal macrosomia, and injuries can occur that harm both the baby and the mother. A baby of this size can also have health problems after birth.

It can be hard to determine if your baby has fetal macrosomia, but your healthcare provider might be able to tell by measuring the fundal height. This is the length from the top of your uterus to the pubic bone. If this height is bigger than normal, your doctor might diagnose your baby with fetal macrosomia.

Polyhydramnios, or excessive amniotic fluid, might also show that your baby has fetal macrosomia. The amniotic fluid that surrounds your baby in the sac represents its urine output, so a larger baby would understandably produce more urine.

Fetal macrosomia can be caused by diabetes—pre-gestational or gestational—in the mother. If you are unable to keep your diabetes under control, it might cause your baby to develop more fat and broader shoulders, which will hinder a vaginal delivery.

If there is a history of fetal macrosomia in your family or if you were born weighing more than eight pounds, thirteen ounces, then it is more likely that your baby will be born larger as well. If you have had one baby with fetal macrosomia, you are more likely to have it happen again in future pregnancies. If you have had several previous pregnancies, even if the babies were born without fetal macrosomia, your likelihood of having a larger baby increases.

Obesity in the mother can also cause fetal macrosomia. Even if you are not overweight before pregnancy, if you gain too much while pregnant, your baby might also gain too much weight too quickly. You are also at an increased risk for giving birth to a baby with fetal macrosomia if you are over thirty-five, or if you go two weeks or longer past your due date.

Maternal risks of fetal macrosomia include difficulty giving birth, damage to the vaginal canal tissues and muscles while giving birth naturally, and bleeding after delivery because your muscles cannot contract back to normal. If you have previously had a c-section or other uterine surgery, fetal macrosomia also puts you at risk for a uterine rupture. This is when you tear open the scar line of your previous surgery. A c-section can prevent this rare event from happening.

Myths About PCOS

Now that you have so much background information about PCOS, the causes, the symptoms, and the treatments, you might have questions about some of the myths you might have heard about PCOS.

PCOS is a Rare Condition

PCOS is far from a rare condition. Though it can only affect women, it affects over one hundred million women worldwide, and five to ten percent of all women in the United States. To break it down further, one in ten women of childbearing age are diagnosed with PCOS. It is the most common hormonal disorder in women of reproductive age.

Many women have PCOS but do not even find out for years because it can be so hard to diagnose. Studies have shown that almost one half of women with PCOS remain undiagnosed, which means millions of women are unaware of their condition and do not know how they can manage their symptoms before they get more severe.

You Did Something to Cause PCOS

It is hard to pinpoint the exact cause of PCOS because many women have different symptoms at the start, but PCOS is never a woman's fault. PCOS is a hormonal condition that might be triggered by an imbalance in male hormones, insulin resistance, and weight. Though you can try to manage the symptoms yourself, you cannot cure PCOS, just like how nothing you did caused it. It is an independent condition that you have to live with once you are diagnosed. Even though you did not cause the condition, you will want to research the disorder so you can be as informed as possible about the symptoms, management, possible complications, and treatments available to you.

You Cannot Get Pregnant If You Have PCOS

PCOS can make it hard to get pregnant, because the condition causes a hormone imbalance. Male hormones are very prevalent in women with PCOS, which understandably makes it harder to have a regular menstrual cycle and routine ovulation. There are natural ways you can try to regulate your period and promote ovulation, with a change in diet, exercise, and supplements. You can also take medication to balance your hormones and increase ovulation, even causing your body to release multiple eggs a month.

If you try different lifestyle changes and medications and still cannot manage to get pregnant naturally, there are other assisted reproductive technologies you can try so you can have a baby. We will explore those options more in depth in a later chapter.

PCOS Symptoms End at Menopause

Because PCOS is a hormonal condition, a common myth is that symptoms will end at menopause, when a woman's hormones change even more. Menopause can change the PCOS symptoms you experience because your estrogen and testosterone levels will change, but it will not cure anything.

As you get older, you will naturally start producing less of the female hormones like estrogen and progesterone. As these hormones decrease, in a period called perimenopause, your period will be less consistent because you are not ovulating anymore. Once you have gone a year without a period, you are categorized as being menopausal. Women diagnosed with PCOS typically reach menopause a year or two later than women without PCOS symptoms.

There are some shared symptoms between PCOS and perimenopause, such as:

- irregular or missed periods
- mood swings
- infertility
- trouble sleeping
- hair loss
- excessive hair growth
- weight gain

If the PCOS symptoms you suffer from are not on this list, it does not mean that you will not experience them in perimenopause and beyond. This list only covers symptoms that PCOS and perimenopause have in common, to show that menopausal hormone changes might not affect your condition.

Perimenopause will bring about other symptoms, like hot flashes and night sweats. This is another symptom that cannot be cured, so it is best to dress in layers, keep your house cool, and avoid caffeine and alcohol.

Many of the approaches to manage PCOS symptoms in your younger years will also apply during perimenopause and menopause. This includes managing your weight by exercising and choosing healthy meal options. You also need to get quality sleep and take care of your mental and emotional health. If natural methods do not help ease your symptoms, you can ask your doctor about medication to manage both your PCOS and perimenopause symptoms. Even once you have gone through menopause, you will still need to maintain a healthy lifestyle to keep your PCOS in check. You should still be aware of the possibility of high blood pressure, high cholesterol, type 2 diabetes, and the health concerns those conditions can cause.

Losing Weight Stops PCOS Symptoms

It is a myth that only overweight women develop PCOS, but there does seem to be a link between weight and the condition. Losing five to ten percent of your body weight can help manage your PCOS symptoms, but it does not completely stop or cure them. If you start exercising regularly and eat a healthy diet but still find yourself unable to lose weight, consult with your doctor to find a solution that might work for you.

Medications may make weight loss easier. Some of the medications discussed in the treatments section will help you lose weight, while also helping to keep some of the other PCOS symptoms in check. Medications that help balance hormone levels or improve your insulin resistance can also benefit your body when it comes to losing weight.

If diet, exercise, and even medications have not helped you lose enough weight to manage your PCOS symptoms or get pregnant, if that is your goal, then you might want to consider weight loss surgery. It is a drastic and invasive procedure, but the benefits are immense. Losing weight this way can help regulate your menstrual cycle, promote ovulation, decrease your odds of developing diabetes and cardiovascular problems, and more. Let us take this time to dive more deeply into weight loss and how it can help you manage your PCOS symptoms.

Chapter 3:

Your Weight and PCOS

Almost half of all women diagnosed with PCOS are overweight, though doctors are not sure if the women are overweight because of PCOS, or if they have PCOS because they are overweight. It is a vicious cycle, but having an ideal weight for your height and body type is important for your overall health, whether you have PCOS or not.

Losing even five to ten percent of your body weight cuts your risk for many severe diseases, but it can also make you feel better. When it comes to PCOS, your mental health is just as important as your physical health, so when something can benefit both of those aspects, you know it is something you need to focus on.

Integrating healthy habits into your existing lifestyle will easily help you keep your weight under control. Start by changing your diet. Eat a diet that is high in fiber, and low in sugar. Eat a lot of fruits, vegetables, and whole grains. Do not eat processed foods, and make sure you are eating good fats. These steps will help you keep your blood sugar levels in check, which not only helps you lose weight, but can also keep you healthy enough to not become diabetic.

Instead of eating three large meals every day, eat four to six small meals throughout the day. It might seem like you are eating more, period, but that is not it. Eating this way will help control your blood sugar levels. In chapter five there are some recipes to help you introduce more healthy meals to your diet, but there are also a few sample meal plans you can reference. These meal plans give you six small meals throughout the day, but we call the additional meals 'snacks.' It might help you adjust to the new diet to think that you are still eating your three square meals, just with different foods than you used to eat. And you are adding in three small snacks as healthy options to balance out any hunger you feel throughout the day.

Exercise for at least thirty minutes a day. Every day. It does not have to be a full-on workout at the gym, but you need to be active every day. You will learn some good exercises for weight loss later in this chapter. In chapter four, you will revisit physical activity for managing PCOS symptoms and learn a few more ways you can add daily exercise.

You might think you need a day off from exercising or a cheat day for your diet, but you do not. You will see the recipes included later and realize that you can still eat delicious meals and snacks—even desserts—so you will not even need to cheat. As far as days off from exercising, that is a no go. Unless you are ill, you do not need to take time off. Thirty minutes a day is nothing. If you exercised too much yesterday, just do a low key exercise routine today. Do not take the day off because it will be that much harder to get back to it. Keep going, stick with the habit, just change up the details of the exercise you are actually doing.

While you are on a quest to lose weight, you will also want to work with your doctor to track your cholesterol and blood pressure levels. As you make changes to your diet, your levels might change, so your doctor should be aware. Monitoring your levels can notify you if a certain diet is not working for you, or can give you a nice boost if you see a major change and realize you are on the right path.

Weight and PCOS

Women who have been diagnosed with PCOS have found that losing ten percent of their body weight has made their periods come back to a regulated cycle. Even minor weight loss can improve insulin sensitivity, which will cut down your risk of heart disease, diabetes, and the other PCOS complications we have discussed previously.

The next time you visit your doctor, mention that you want to lose weight to help manage your PCOS symptoms. The doctor will check your weight, waist size, and body mass index. Body mass index, also called BMI, is the ratio of your height to your weight. Checking this, along with your waist size, will help the doctor see how your weight is distributed. If you are overweight but have a small waist, your weight might be going to your legs or buttocks, so you will need to approach losing that weight differently than the weight around your waist. Most women with PCOS have weight around their waists because of the way hormones and insulin resistance affect belly fat. But the doctor will take all of this into consideration before helping you lose weight.

Your doctor might first recommend that you change your diet and add in physical activity to kickstart your weight loss. However, since you have already been doing your own research, you know this information and have already started taking those measures. Tell your doctor this so they know you have already been making changes and are ready to step it up.

Medication can be prescribed to help women with PCOS lose weight. Several medications that are approved for weight loss also help manage PCOS symptoms, such as birth control pills, anti-androgen medications, and metformin. Some research has found that these medications can help obese women with PCOS lose weight because they change the way your body uses insulin, and also reduce testosterone production.

Insulin is a hormone that helps the cells in your body convert sugar from your bloodstream into energy your body will use later. If you have insulin resistance, as women with PCOS have, the cells in your organs, muscles, and other tissues do not absorb your blood sugar the way they should. As a result, you might be diagnosed as diabetic because you have too much sugar in your bloodstream. This extra sugar can also cause you to put on weight even if you feel like you are eating a regular diet. Insulin resistance also makes you crave sugar, so if you give in to these cravings more than you realize, you will definitely end up putting on weight.

Weight Loss

Exercise is a great way to increase your potential for weight loss. Diet plays a big part in weight loss, but we will get to that in a later chapter.

Cardio

Studies have been done on women with PCOS who work out, and researchers found that doing forty-five to sixty minutes of cardio three times each week cuts body fat by over four percent! Losing this much fat will also improve your sensitivity to insulin, which in turn can keep some of your other symptoms in check.

Cardio is any exercise that raises your heart rate, increases your breathing, and improves the functions of your lungs, heart, and circulatory system. People most commonly think of cardio as any sustained exercise, like jogging. Walking on a treadmill is great exercise, but unless you crank up the speed of the treadmill, it does not count as cardio.

That does not mean that cardio has to be done at the gym! You can jog around your neighborhood, do aerobic exercise videos in your bedroom, practice strenuous dance routines, or jump rope for longer than twenty minutes. You can ride your bike or run stairs. Even raking leaves or shoveling snow can be a cardio exercise if you put your all into it and work for a longer time without stopping.

If you cannot work out briskly for twenty minutes or more, consider trying high-intensity interval training, or HIIT. HIIT is a method of exercise that breaks up brief periods of intense exercise with even shorter recovery periods. The main idea is to do a crazy workout for a minute or two until you think you cannot do any more. A brief rest brings you much-needed relief, but also lets your body feel that rush of adrenaline that makes it say, "Oh, I can do that! Let me try again." So you do the exercise again until you feel like you cannot, and then you rest again.

It might sound like a form of torture, I know, but once you try it out you might find you love it. The workout itself rarely lasts for thirty minutes, so you get it done quickly but feel a major impact because the exercise was so strenuous. Some studies have shown that HIIT does not effectively improve obesity, but it does reduce your body's fat mass as a whole, so it is worth a try to at least get in the swing of exercising. If it does not seem to be working for you, you can change to a different type of exercise but know that you tried HIIT and used it to get your body in gear!

If you go to the gym, you will have more options for cardio workouts, including swimming, kickboxing, or attending classes that would help you stick to a schedule. A lot of women with PCOS have found that going to classes holds them accountable, not to mention you have a group of women there cheering you on!

If you would rather do cardio at home but do not want to bike, jump rope, or go out for a run, look for videos online. There are a lot of choices for at-home cardio workouts that you can do on your own or with a few props. You can also try different videos to see what host you like, and see how long each workout routine lasts. The best part of doing cardio at home is that you can find something that best fits your schedule, space, and style of exercise.

Keep in mind that cardio exercising uses a lot of muscles, usually in your legs, torso, and core. While working your biceps is great, it does not require as much full-body effort as other workouts, so your heart and blood will not get pounding and you will not feel the effect as much as true cardio. Cardio workouts will increase your body's ability to intake oxygen while also pushing it to send blood to your extremities. Taking time to do cardio helps your circulatory system and lungs in the long-term to reach optimal function whether you are working out or relaxing.

Weight Training

Weight training is another good way for women with PCOS to lose weight. A study found that doing weight training three times a week helps you lose belly fat, reduce testosterone, and balance blood sugar levels.

Weight training is a type of exercise that relies on using weight resistance to build muscles. Though the purpose is to strengthen your muscles, weight training does lead to weight loss. This activity is tough to do at home unless you are already an experienced weightlifter. Investing in a weight bench and weights is very expensive, and it is not recommended that you lift weights without a spotter. If you lift weights at a gym, you can have someone nearby to help you if needed, or you can even work with a personal trainer.

Some minor weight training can be done at home if you have hand weights or ankle weights. You can strap on ankle weights and wear them while you bike, walk, jog, or jump rope. You can also hold hand weights for extra resistance while walking or jogging. It might not sound like much, but you are so used to walking around with just yourself that carrying a little extra resistant weight will make a difference in your fitness over time.

Yoga

Yoga is a great exercise to take up if you have PCOS. Not only will yoga help you lose weight and stay flexible and healthy, but it is also a very calming yet active hobby that can help you practice self-care. Once you start practicing yoga, you will find yourself coming back to certain poses when you feel stressed or upset. The pose will calm you, allow you to get back in touch with your physical body, and help you feel energized and strong.

A recent study found that women who practiced yoga for one hour three times a week saw their testosterone levels decrease by twenty-nine percent over several months (Patel et al., 2020). This is an amazing benefit, as yoga alone can make your body stronger and able to reach a different plane of relaxation, while also helping you lose weight.

Just as the root cause of PCOS can be hard to explain, it can be hard to explain the multitude of ways yoga benefits your body—until you start practicing and experience it for yourself. Yoga works deeper than your muscles and your core to relieve stress that has been stored in your body for years. So many of the yoga poses require you to comfortably sink into a pose and hold it while you breathe deeply and let your body ease into the position. Over time you will find yoga to be relaxing.

Yoga postures, also called asanas, often open up your body, including your pelvis, to promote relaxation. When you pair this with purposeful breathing, also called pranayamas, you not only calm your mind but also de-toxify and de-stress your entire system.

Keep in mind that some asanas might require you to put pressure on your abdomen—you do not need to do these poses! A few of these to watch out for include:

- Bow pose
- Boat pose
- Cobra pose
- Superman pose

The whole point of yoga is to do the positions to the best of your ability, but as soon as something is uncomfortable or starts to hurt, you should stop doing it. Not doing certain poses does not make you a failure; in yoga, as with PCOS, knowing the limitations and capabilities of your body is of utmost importance. Yoga is also a great practice that can work for all body types, so do not think that you are too out of shape or not athletic enough to do yoga. Yoga meets you where you are, and you will benefit from it!

You can find yoga routines online or find classes to attend locally. Many yoga teachers post routines online and specify the length of the practice and what the intentions are. This means you can search specifically for yoga for women with PCOS, yoga for weight loss, yoga for flexibility, and more. If you are worried about doing a pose correctly, you might want to start by attending classes where a teacher can help you find the best poses for your body.

It is recommended to stick to gentle poses to help manage your PCOS. You can hold them for a longer period of time, but they do not involve the contortions or rapid movements of some of the other poses. A few specific asanas that women with PCOS have found relaxation in include:

- Butterfly pose
- Reclining butterfly pose
- Bharadvajasana
- Shavasana
- Padma Sadhana
- Chakki Chalanasana
- Sun Salutations

Each of these poses is slow-moving poses that you will hold for several deep breaths, which will ease your body from any daily pain you feel into a mode of aware relaxation. They will bring blood flow to the pelvic region while giving you the chance to practice mindfulness and feel the stretch in your body. You can mention these poses to a teacher if you are attending a yoga class in person, or you can seek out illustrations or videos of the poses online and do them in the privacy of your home.

Beginning Yoga Poses

Here are seven yoga exercises you can try to get the feel for how practicing yoga might help you manage your PCOS symptoms. These poses have been specifically chosen for women with PCOS.

Breathing Exercise

Let us start with a breathing exercise that you can do to get in the right mindset to practice yoga. This exercise alone will help the stress melt away from your shoulders so you feel more relaxed. This technique is called Kapalbhati Pranayama, and has been shown to help women with PCOS manage their weight, blood sugar levels, along with stress levels.

Start with an empty stomach, because you will be using your abdominal muscles to exhale forcefully.

Sit tall in a firm chair or sit cross-legged in an open space on the floor.

Close your eyes and start relaxing your entire body.

Inhale deeply through your nostrils while noticing the expansion in your chest.

Use your abdominal muscles to forcefully exhale.

Repeat ten times to complete a cycle. This might take you as long as five minutes while you adjust to the practice. You should feel your abdominal muscles contracting with each exhale.

Bow Pose

The bow pose, also called Dhanurasana, helps relieve menstrual pain, stimulates circulation to your reproductive organs, and helps to regulate your menstrual flow. The gentle stretching releases tension from your abdomen and stretches the neck, shoulders, and legs muscles. This full-body stretch is a great option to release stress from your muscles to achieve relaxation.

Start by lying down flat on your stomach. Stretch your arms down the sides of your body.

Slowly fold your knees up and reach down so your hands can grab your ankles. If you cannot grab both ankles at the same time, do each leg individually. Keep practicing up, and you will be proud when you reach the point where you can grab both ankles at the same time!

Take a deep breath in while you lift your chest up off the ground. As your chest lifts, keep pulling your legs up. Breathe out as you pull.

Hold the bow pose for fifteen seconds, and breathe steadily while you focus on how your body feels as it stretches.

To release your body from the bow pose, slowly let your chest and legs ease back toward the ground.

Release the hold on your ankles, and ease them to the ground—do not let them thud back down into place.

Take a minute to relax on the ground in your original pose, face down.

Repeat this pose three times to complete a cycle.

Garland Pose

The garland pose, also called malasana, works to strengthen your pelvic floor and abdominal core while inspiring your hips to widen. This pose increases blood flow and circulation to your pelvic region, aids your digestion, and improves your metabolism.

If you have yoga blocks, you can use them to sit on for additional support until you become experienced with this pose. You can also use a firm cushion if you do not have yoga blocks.

Stand with your feet shoulder's width apart.

Bend your knees and lower your buttocks as you slowly sink into a squatting position.

Bring your hands to your chest in a prayer position, also called anjali mudra. Let your thumbs touch your chest bone to keep your chest lifted and feel your heart beat beneath your hands.

Press your upper arms against the inside of your knees. Focus on your body so you can keep it in position with your spine straight. Let your elbows press into your knees to widen the hips.

Extend your lower back and pull your shoulder blades back towards one another.

Stay in this position while you take five long, deep, relaxing breaths.

Come out of the position by slowly straightening your legs until you return to standing position.

Repeat the garland pose a total of three times to complete a cycle.

Bridge Pose

The bridge pose, also called Setu Bandhasana, calms your brain down and reduces the stress and anxiety you feel. It also relieves any tension you are holding in your back muscles.

Start by lying flat on your back. Fold your knees and place your feet hip-width apart on the flood.

Place your hands palm down on either side of your body.

Take a deep breath while you slowly lift your first lower back, then mid-back, and then upper back up off the floor.

As your pelvis lifts up, feel your torso lengthen and strengthen from your pelvis, all the way to your sternum.

Roll your shoulders back gently and slowly bring your chest up toward your chin.

Keep your thighs parallel both to each other and to the floor. Feel the entire bottom of your feet press firmly into the ground. Your feet should feel strong, like the foundation of this stance, even though you are lying down.

Breathe slowly and deeply, counting your breaths as you stay in this pose for one or two minutes.

Repeat up this pose five times to complete the cycle.

Head-to-Knee Pose

The head-to-knee pose is also called Janusirsana. This is a great pose to awaken your entire body.

Sit on your yoga mat. If you do not have a yoga mat, you can spread a beach towel out on a rug or carpeted surface.

Stretch your left leg to the far corner of your mat or towel. If you are sitting on the floor without a mat or towel, gently stretch your left leg as far forward and slightly to the left as you can.

Keep your foot flexed with the back of your heel pushing down into the ground. Let your toes point to the sky.

Bend your right knee and keep your right foot tucked as closely to your pelvic region as you are comfortable with.

Stretch your arms out over your legs and breathe in deeply.

When you exhale, move your upper body gently forward towards your left foot, while slowly swooping your right arm up in a graceful arc over your head.

You will feel a strong stretch and twist in your torso. Your shoulders and hips will feel wider and more open, which will give a gentle massage to those joints.

This exercise asks for purposeful breathing in time with your stretches and movements. As you breathe, you should feel your chest and core expanding and contracting.

Do the head-to-knee pose eight times on each side.

Cat-Cow Pose

The cat-cow pose is also called the Chakravakasana. It is a slightly more advanced pose, and if you read through it but are unsure how the asana should look, you can find a video online to make sure you do it correctly.

Start in the tabletop position. This is when your body basically looks like a table because you are on your hands and knees. Keep your palms flat on the ground with your wrists and elbows aligned beneath your shoulders. Keep your knees under your hips, and your ankles should be straight back from your knees.

You can curl your toes under or keep the tops of your feet down on the mat, depending on what feels most comfortable for you. This may change as you hold the pose.

Take a deep breath and bend your elbows. Lower your belly as you lift your chin and tailbone at the same time. You should feel each of your vertebrae in your spinal column moving like a wave.

Reverse the pose as you exhale. Start by tucking your tailbone and chin back in. Arch your back as you pull your navel towards your spine. While you do this, your chin will naturally tip back down towards your chest.

As this pose is slow and gentle, you can repeat it as many times as you would like to relax and de-stress.

Butterfly Pose

The butterfly pose is also called the bound angle pose, or Supta Baddha Konasana. This asana is great for your spine and back, but also helps you release tension from your shoulders.

If this pose seems too difficult at first, you can modify it by using folded blankets or pillows under your shoulders, under your head at a slight incline, and under your thighs.

Start by sitting on your yoga mat (or a towel, or just a stretch of carpeted floor). Stretch your legs straight out in front of you.

Bend both knees and bring your heels in towards your body and press the soles of your feet together. Your knees will naturally drop to the sides as you do this. Make sure they fall gracefully, and not with a thump.

Lean backwards until your back touches the floor. Keep your arms open with your palms facing up towards the sky.

Close your eyes and inhale and exhale deeply for three to five minutes. If you feel comfortable, you can hold this pose longer and use it as a mindfulness exercise to practice purposeful breathing and relaxation.

When you are ready to come out of the pose, do so slowly and gently. Roll onto your right side and pause in that position for a few deep breaths. Push back up to your seated position and center yourself with a few deep breaths.

Why It Is Hard to Lose Weight With PCOS

Most women struggle with their weight for their entire lives. It is just a common thing we have to deal with, like it or not. But women who are diagnosed with PCOS not only struggle with weight gain, but also have trouble losing weight, even if they are eating a healthy diet and exercising regularly.

No matter what the cause, weight gain can be detrimental to your health. Women with PCOS are more likely to develop many of the severe complications associated with weight gain and insulin resistance, including:

- Infertility
- High cholesterol
- High blood pressure
- Type 2 diabetes
- Sleep apnea
- Endometrial cancer
- Heart disease

Women with PCOS have insulin resistance, which not only causes them to gain weight due to trouble converting sugar to energy, but also prevents them from losing weight because their body thinks they need the sugar, so they pack it on. This sugar typically manifests as weight around a woman's waist, which makes it even harder to lose. Abdominal fat is the most dangerous kind of fat because it can cause an elevated risk of heart disease and other severe health conditions.

Another side effect of insulin resistance is that high insulin levels increase the levels of male hormones. High androgen and testosterone levels cause weight gain, typically also only in the abdomen, just like with insulin resistance.

Insulin resistance also makes women feel hungrier. They crave sugar because their body thinks they are not getting enough. The insulin levels are so out of order that, even while the body is packing on pounds because it cannot convert sugar to energy, it is demanding more and more. Appetite regulating hormones like cholecystokinin, ghrelin, and leptin also do not occur at normal levels in women with PCOS, so it is harder to know when you are full and should stop eating.

Chapter 4:

Changing Your Lifestyle for PCOS

Since there is no cure for PCOS, changing your lifestyle is the most effective way to manage your symptoms. Medications can be a supplementary action, but you do not want to depend on them too much. Making some foundational lifestyle changes might help you manage your symptoms enough that you do not need medication. Or if you would still like to use medication, you will already have made some changes so your doctor can be sure to prescribe the exact right medicine to manage the rest of your symptoms.

Eating a healthy and balanced diet, being physically active and exercising, sleeping well, and practicing self-care to manage your stress can help balance out your hormones that PCOS has imbalanced.

Not only does changing your lifestyle help manage your PCOS symptoms, but it also helps you prevent these symptoms from becoming more severe in time. Taking control of your life now might keep you from having complications when you get older.

Managing PCOS with Lifestyle

Changing your diet is a huge lifestyle change, but the recipes and meal plans in chapter five will help you ease into that change. Hopefully you have been integrating more exercise into your lifestyle after going through the weight loss chapter. But the process does not end there. Other lifestyle changes you need to make include sleep, stress, self-care, and more.

If you smoke, find a way that will help you quit. Go cold turkey if you are brave, or get the patch or gum if you need to step down over time. Smoking is bad for your health, period, but it can really exacerbate PCOS symptoms to a painful degree. Smoking, in conjunction with some of the hormone levels PCOS causes in women can, can lead to very severe complications and diseases down the line. Quit now, while you are making so many other lifestyle changes. Your body will thank you for it.

Alcohol can also exacerbate PCOS symptoms. Drinking excessively is very unhealthy, so you should carefully watch your portions regardless of your PCOS symptoms. But even a little alcohol can cause symptoms to flare unchecked. It is especially important to let your doctor know how much alcohol you drink every week, because it could react badly with some of the medications and supplements you might choose to take to manage PCOS.

Physical Activity

In addition to the major physical activities we introduced in chapter three, specifically cardio, weight training, and yoga, you can also easily introduce other physical activity into your daily life. Being active is an important part of managing PCOS symptoms. Physical activity has been proven to alleviate symptoms and reduce the risk of them becoming more severe, resulting in long-term health complications.

There are many benefits of regular physical activity for women with PCOS, including:

- increased energy levels
- reduced insulin resistance
- improved menstrual regularity
- increased fertility and ovulation
- reduced anxiety and depression
- easier ongoing weight maintenance

Studies have shown that any type of physical activity, whether moderate or vigorous, can effectively improve PCOS symptoms. Women with PCOS who want to lose a moderate amount of weight will want to aim for thirty minutes of physical activity a day. At least two days a week should include weight training to help strengthen your muscles, but for the rest of it, any moderate to vigorous aerobic activity will help lose the most weight.

Women diagnosed with PCOS who want to prevent weight gain or maintain their weight should do at least two and a half hours of moderate physical activity a week, or an hour and a half of vigorous exercise. Spaced out over a week, this equals about twenty minutes of moderate activity a day, or fifteen minutes of vigorous exercise a day. When you break it down like that, you can see how easily physical activity can fit into your daily life.

Walking

Walking briskly can get your heart rate going and be a form of cardio, but even if you do not push your walking pace to rival a full-blown workout, walking can be a great physical activity to help manage your PCOS symptoms.

Instead of sitting for extended periods of time, make sure you get up and walk around. Take the long way to go to the bathroom or the break room at work. Or instead of sneaking to the break room for a snack, just go on a walk! Your mind will thank you for taking a moment to get outside of your work environment, and your body will thank you for the extra steps you are taking.

If you live close enough to places like neighborhood stores, coffee shops, restaurants, or even your workplace, consider walking every so often. You do not have to give up your car completely, but the additional steps will do wonders for your health.

You might be someone who works better if you can see concrete progress, so consider getting a pedometer or a smartwatch that can keep track of your steps. You can set goals and push yourself to exceed them every day. Many of those technologies also convert your steps into calories lost, so you will get to see the real difference steps can make on your health.

Walking is enough physical activity that it will help improve your mood and alleviate stress and anxiety, but you can also make it a social event. Walk with your neighbors in the evening after dinner and catch up on your day while you get some exercise. Walk during your lunch break with your favorite coworker and relieve some work stress during the day. Meet friends at the park and walk around the track while you plan a surprise party. Making your walk a social endeavor is a win-win situation: you will get the mental and emotional benefits of catching up with your friends, and you will be distracted from the fact that you are actually exercising while doing so!

Squatting

It sounds crazy, but squatting is actually a great exercise to help you increase your strength and work to lose weight. Squats work the biggest groups of muscles in your body, like your core, back, glutes, and quads. You are already squatting when you sit down and standing up from sitting, so why not add just enough to make it an exercise?

Stand tall and strong with your feet firmly on the ground beneath your shoulders. Take a deep breath and start lowering your body down like you are going to sit on a chair. Keep your back straight and your chest up because this engages your core muscles. Keep lowering your body until your thighs are parallel to the ground. If you can go lower, by all means work those muscles! Exhale while you keep your core tight and engaged. Try to hold this pose for at least one additional inhale and exhale, then use your muscles to slowly pull your body back up to a standing position.

If you want to step up your squatting game, add some hand weights to the exercise outlined above! The weights will provide extra resistance to the motions.

Push Ups

Push ups might seem hard to do if you are not athletic or used to exercising because they require a lot of upper body strength. That strength can be hard to cultivate since most of us are so used to more sedentary lifestyles due to our work. But doing push ups is a great way to start developing that upper body strength, even if your end goal is not to get bodybuilder muscles.

In addition to requiring upper body strength and helping to develop your biceps, push ups also work your glutes, legs, and core muscles.

Put your palms flat on the floor, slightly wider than your shoulders. Tighten your core muscles so you can keep your torso straight. Stretch your legs back and keep them tightly pressed together, including your feet. Take a deep breath and move your arms so your body lowers to the ground. Keep your core muscles tight as you lower your body, and tuck your elbows back to your sides. Exhale your breath as you push your body back up to your starting position. Push yourself to do as many push ups as you can in one round. The next time you exercise, push yourself to do more push ups. Keep challenging yourself to do even one more push up so you know you are getting stronger.

Food

The next chapter is all about your PCOS diet, what foods you need to add to and remove from your diet, and three set diets that have helped women with PCOS in the past. There are also recipes and meal plan suggestions to follow. So you will get to learn all of those details very soon. For now, let us touch on why food is so important to women with PCOS.

When you make changes to your food intake, make sure they are changes you can keep up for a long time. Fad diets often do more harm than good, so do not try to lose weight using an unproven diet. The three you will learn about later have been proven to be effective and have research to back them up, as well as testimonials from women with PCOS who have followed the diets. But any diet that claims to help you lose twenty pounds in five days is going to be an unsustainable fad diet you do not want to fall for.

A lot of women have emotional relationships with food, and it can be hard to identify those patterns and change them for the better. It is easiest to be honest with yourself and your feelings towards food. Everyone has a comfort food that makes them feel cozy after a hard day, but if you are justifying every indulgence as a necessary comfort food, you need to admit that to yourself.

Sometimes you might eat because you are bored. If there is nothing else to do, why not make a snack and eat it? If you are not hungry, you do not need to eat the snack. Instead, you could read a book or put away the laundry or do another chore you have been putting off. You might eat because you are lonely, but instead of eating, why not call or text a friend? Send an email, write a letter, reach out to someone instead of eating. The same goes for sadness, or happiness, or celebrating a raise at work, or mourning a loss. Instead of eating to ignore your feelings, sit and feel your feelings. Acknowledge why you are feeling them and how you can move past them. Keep yourself busy in other ways that do not involve food.

It also helps if you can admit when you are hungry and when you are just craving something. Commercials and social media ads are way too good at making you think you need an ice-cold soda or that perfectly made hamburger even though you just ate dinner an hour ago. A healthy, completely manageable step to take is to stop and think before you eat. Do you really need to get into your car and go through a drive-thru at ten o'clock at night if you just cooked a delicious dinner and should be getting into bed? No way! Do the burger and soda look like the absolute best meal on the planet? Oh yeah. But you do not need them. You are not hungry. It is not a healthy choice even if you were hungry. And, let us be honest, would your burger look like that? Doubtful. It probably would not taste that great, either. And then you would have feelings of guilt to beat yourself up over because you splurged on a meal you did not even want.

Identify any triggers you have regarding food, and work on finding the root cause of each of them. Once that is done, you should be able to have a better relationship with food. And, now that you have laid the groundwork, you are ready to shift your food choices to be much healthier than they might have been in the past.

A simple step you can take is to decrease Advanced Glycation End products (AGEs) that are created when foods are cooked at high temperatures. Scientifically speaking, they are compounds formed when glucose binds with proteins. Since women with PCOS already have problems processing glucose, AGEs can be detrimental when it comes to losing weight and keeping it off.

Researchers also believe that AGEs contribute to certain degenerative diseases and aging. Paired with possible complications from PCOS symptoms, this is not a good mix. Fortunately, cutting down on AGEs has been shown to significantly reduce insulin levels in women with PCOS.

Foods high in AGEs include foods that come from animals and are high in fat and protein. Processed foods are also high in AGEs, along with certain cheeses, eggs, butter, cream cheese, and mayonnaise. Applying high heat increases AGE levels, like when you grill, fry, roast, sauté, sear, and boil foods.

Some simple healthy food choices you can start making even before getting lost in the diets and recipes to come include:

- using healthy cooking oils, like olive oil or canola oil
- steaming or baking food instead of frying
- drinking water instead of soda or juice
- balancing meals to have protein, vegetables, and whole grains
- serving correct portions of each aspect of your meal
- eating high fiber cereals and grains
- adding beans, lentils, and chickpeas in your diet for more fiber and to keep you feeling full
- eating raw, unsalted nuts as a filling snack
- eating more fish, especially salmon
- eating only when you are hungry
- stopping when you feel full

Changing your relationship with food now can help prevent you from putting on more weight from this point on. You might still have weight you need to lose, but if you start seeing food differently right now, you are already taking action that will positively impact you in the future. Keeping yourself from gaining weight is an amazing way to keep your PCOS symptoms in check.

Sleep

Women with PCOS suffer from sleep problems. Sleep apnea is a disorder we have previously discussed. Sleep apnea causes you to stop breathing for brief periods in your sleep. It messes up your body's oxygen flow and disrupts your sleep cycle. Because it messes up your body's oxygen supply, sleep apnea can cause further complications, like high blood pressure, lower pain tolerance, heart disease, weight problems, and mood swings.

Symptoms of sleep apnea include:
- having a sore throat in the mornings
- feeling very tired during the daytime
- having trouble focusing on your daytime activities
- loud, uneven, disruptive snoring when you are asleep
- periods where you stop breathing while you are asleep

If you are having any of these symptoms, either that you notice or that your partner notices, inform your doctor. If you are diagnosed with sleep apnea, there are breathing treatments you can use while you sleep, like a CPAP machine, to keep your breathing steady. You can try alternatives to the CPAP machine, such as other oral appliances, nasal valve therapy, bilevel positive airway pressure (BiPAP), or even surgery.

Women with PCOS should aim to get eight to ten hours of sleep a night, even if you think you can get away with six to seven hours. Aiming for this amount of sleep does not mean you will actually get that much, but it is a good goal, and it can be something you get closer and closer to with practice. A lot of women with PCOS suffer from insomnia, but developing a bedtime routine and practicing good sleep hygiene can help you change your sleep habits, which might in turn eliminate your insomnia.

Of course, you know first-hand what the power of a good night's sleep can do for you throughout the day. So, focusing on developing techniques that will result in a more restful sleep could drastically improve your mental, emotional and physical wellbeing.

Sleep Hygiene

Good sleep hygiene includes keeping your bedroom as neat as you can. If you have enough space in your living quarters to use your bedroom only for sleeping, you should do that. Read and watch shows in the living room, eat in the kitchen, and keep your bedroom just for sleeping. This means that when you enter that room, your mind and body will already know that it is time to prepare for sleep. If you use your bedroom to read in bed, or sit on your bed and have snacks, it will be harder to associate this space with sleep, and it will be harder for you to fall asleep once you are in your bed because you are using it for other things.

Sleep hygiene can also include developing a bedtime routine. Do not eat any food, especially fatty foods, close to bedtime. Your body does not digest food when you are sleeping, so it could harm all the work you have been putting into weight loss and weight management. Eating before bed might also make it harder for you to breathe if you have sleep apnea or other struggles while you sleep. You will also want to avoid caffeinated drinks, though a warm tea with no caffeine might help you unwind before bed.

Put your phone down an hour before you want to go to sleep. Stop watching a show or doing anything with a screen so you give your eyes and mind time to relax. A warm bath is a nice way to wind down at the end of the day. You can also do a slow, peaceful yoga routine—there are actually online video routines created specifically to prepare you for a good night's sleep.

You might make time to read a few pages of a book before bedtime. This exercises your mind in a different way, while still making it tired. Make sure you are reading a physical book, not looking at an eBook on a screen! There is nothing wrong with digital books during the day, but avoiding screens near bedtime is a crucial step in promoting good sleep habits. White noise machines might help you fall asleep and stay asleep, or soft calming music.

Other things you may want to try to get to sleep quickly and stay asleep longer include regulating your breath. Just as this is an important aspect of yoga, it can also make a difference in your sleep patterns. Exhale through your mouth completely, until you feel your lungs deflate. Close your mouth and inhale through your nose as you count to four. Hold your breath and count to seven. Open your mouth to exhale completely while you count to eight. If you repeat this technique a few times, it will calm you down and relax your body for sleep.

You might be struggling to go to sleep because you have so much on your mind. Take some time before bed to think about your day. Go over the tough things you experienced, and resolve anything you let bother you. Think about what you need to accomplish tomorrow, but do not let it cause anxiety. Just think about it and let the thoughts go. You can also write them down if you think that will help you get them out of your head. You can write a nightly journal entry, or just make a list of things that happened or things you still need to do. Any way to prevent these thoughts from circling through your mind all night on constant repeat will be beneficial to your sleep cycle.

Having something on your mind is not always a bad thing, as long as your thoughts are not stressful.

Sometimes thinking happy thoughts can relax your brain to the point where it eases into sleep quickly. Thinking good thoughts can also calm your brain enough that you can have peaceful sleep all night long, with no negativity entering your dreams and startling you awake.

Sometimes just trying to stay awake can make you sleepier. You are in your bed, in a dark room, and you are trying to convince yourself to stay away. On a normal night, you might have anxious thoughts scrolling through your mind nonstop, but it seems like as soon as you focus enough to try and stay awake, those thoughts float away and you are grasping at straws, trying to think any thought that can keep you alert. Instead, your mind cannot settle on anything so it starts to shut down, your eyes start to close, and before you know it, you are asleep.

Find the ideal temperature for sleeping. Most people's bodies get cooler throughout the night, so you might be waking up because you get too cold. You might want to turn up the heat before you go to bed. You can also keep an extra blanket within reach and add a layer before you go to sleep or when you feel cool. This means if you feel warmer at night, you can take off the extra blanket. Because some women also have trouble sleeping if they are too warm, you want to be sure to find the perfect temperature balance for your body.

If you can get away with not having a clock in your bedroom, you should keep it out. Or position it far enough away from the bed that you can hear the alarm but not see the time. If you do wake up in the middle of the night, you might be able to roll over and get back to sleep on your own, but if your eyes immediately find the clock, you are more likely to wake up. Then you might start calculating how long you have left to sleep before you have to get up and start your day. And that time keeps getting shorter and shorter, which frustrates you and keeps you from getting back to sleep even more. It is a struggle we have all experienced, but that is just how our brains work. If you cannot have a clock, keep the clock face out of sight, or use your phone face down as an alarm, you might be able to prevent this disruption from occurring.

Do you take naps during the day? If you are so tired from not sleeping all night, you might be compelled to nap after lunch or after a long day at work. These naps throw off your sleep schedule, so try to avoid them if you can. Short naps might be necessary to shake off your grogginess and increase your focus, but unless you set an alarm and actually get up when it goes off, naps typically stretch to an hour or two.

If you are sick and need to rest, by all means you should take a nap! There is a difference between a nap "just because" or a nap for self-care, and your body will let you know which is which. If you are feeling tired because you did not sleep well the night before, push through your day and go to bed early. Going to bed early a few nights might help you get on a sleep schedule that allows you even more hours of quality sleep.

You might not be active enough during the day if you frequently find yourself unable to fall asleep. You do not have to wear yourself out every day, but feeling exhausted does help you get to sleep. Since increasing your physical activity is a way to manage your PCOS and, it turns out, also helps you improve the quality of your sleep, it is a no-brainer that this is a lifestyle change you should make for all of the benefits it brings you.

Make sure your mattress and pillow are comfortable. You might be experiencing bad sleep because your body cannot get comfortable. If you have a good mattress and pillow, you might want to sprinkle them with lavender oil or use an oil diffuser in your bedroom. Lavender oil has been used in aromatherapy throughout history to promote calmness and inspire peaceful sleep.

Supplements

If you try all of these natural ways to get to sleep and stay asleep through the night, you might want to try sleep supplements. Some sleep supplements encourage sleep by boosting your body's production of sleep-promoting hormones or by calming brain activity.

Melatonin helps your body naturally instigate a sleep cycle. Your body produces this hormone on its own, but if you take additional doses it can help regulate your sleep. It can also help you stay asleep if you wake often during the night and improve your sleep quality. Take the advised dosage an hour before bed so you give it time to kick in.

Magnesium helps activate the neurons in your brain that are responsible for sleep. Magnesium is found in nuts and leafy greens, so if you add those to your diet then you can naturally elevate your magnesium levels. The supplement should be taken with food, so you can take it with your dinner every evening and be ready for a good night's sleep. Check with your doctor before starting to take magnesium, because the wrong dosage might cause nausea and muscle cramps.

Gamma-aminobutyric acid, or GABA, is a chemical produced in the brain that helps your central nervous system calm down at the end of the day. Taking a supplement of GABA will help kickstart the compound in your brain to initiate your body's sleep response.

The valerian plant has been used as a sleep aid throughout history. Valerian helps raise the levels of GABA your brain produces, and GABA boosts relaxation naturally. Valerian might give you headaches or stomach aches if you take it too frequently, so this might be something you save for those nights when good sleep is crucial. Take the supplement one to two hours before bed, or brew two to three grams of the dried root in a cup of warm water and drink as tea before you go to sleep.

Tart cherry juice is a natural source of melatonin, so sipping a glass of it an hour or two before bed will raise your melatonin levels and prepare you for sleep.

Cannabidiol, or CBD oil, is a compound found in marijuana and hemp plants. It does not have the tetrahydrocannabinol (THC) that will get you high, but CBD oil can help you feel drowsy. It helps people relax and feel calm, and even has been proven to ease anxiety. CBD oil may make you feel nauseous, so start with a low dose and see how it makes you feel before stepping up your dosage.

Glycine is an amino acid that makes a big difference in your sleep. It increases your serotonin levels. Serotonin is a chemical naturally found in your brain that inspires sleep by increasing your blood flow and lowering your body temperature. Take your glycine supplement about an hour before bedtime for best results.

A compound your body makes from the food you eat is 5-hydroxytryptophan, or 5-HTP. Your body uses 5-HTP to produce melatonin, which is an important hormone for sleep. You can take melatonin by itself, as we said before, but taking 5-HTP made from plant seeds might give you a different reaction. If you try melatonin and do not get the results you want, consider trying 5-HTP as a backup.

Practice Self-Care

Eating a healthy diet and exercising are key aspects to managing your PCOS symptoms, but almost equally important is practicing self-care. Stress is a major trigger for PCOS, and it is easy to get stressed since you are trying to balance so much at one time. Self-care might look like different things for different people.

Practicing yoga is a form of self-care for people who enjoy that activity. It calms you and releases stress from your body while also allowing you to focus on something physical, so your mind can relax as well. Exercising is also a form of self-care for people who like to get physical.

If you are not finding peace in yoga or other physical activities, you do not have to push yourself to use it as a form of self-care. Self-care is all about finding what makes you feel better and allowing yourself to enjoy it. This means you immerse yourself fully in the activity, without worrying about what you should be doing, or what you have to do later. Stay in the moment and be content with what you are doing.

Reduce Stress

Exercise is a great way to relieve stress because it lowers your body's stress hormones, like cortisol, while releasing endorphins that make you feel good and naturally improve your mood. Since exercise works your body, it will also make you more tired at the end of the day so you will get better sleep. As you exercise, you will lose weight or maintain your current weight, which will improve your self-esteem. And if you feel good and look good, you will have one less thing to be stressed about. If you enjoy the physical activity you are doing, exercise will not feel like a chore, it will feel fun.

You can take natural supplements to help relieve your stress if some of the other options do not work. Here are a few effective ones:

- Lemon balm. Lemon balm is part of the mint family. Mint has been studied for its years and it has been found to be effective at reducing anxiety.
- Ashwagandha. Ashwagandha is an herb used in Ayurvedic, or holistic, medicine to reduce stress and anxiety.
- Omega-3 fatty acids. Omega-3 fatty acids are found in some fish, which you can add to your diet for anti-anxiety benefits as well as healthy meals. Taking an omega-3 supplement will give you extra doses of this healthy fat and help reduce your feelings of stress.
- Valerian. We mentioned valerian root in the sleep section, but you can also take it to reduce stress. Since it reduces your GABA receptors, it will lower your anxiety. Since this relaxes you, it might be a good idea to keep taking it closer to bedtime.
- Green tea. Green tea is a healthy beverage that you can drink with your balanced diet because you are not adding any sugar or caffeine into your system. Green tea has many antioxidants

that help lower stress and anxiety by boosting your serotonin levels.

As with all of the medications and supplements we have discussed before, these supplements might interact with other medications you are on. They might cause side effects that make your PCOS symptoms more severe, so you will want to talk with your doctor before you start taking any of these.

Aromatherapy is a nice way to relieve stress. You can get an oil diffuser to help the scent flow through your house, or you might want to use scented candles. You can even dilute essential oils in a carrier oil, like coconut oil, and apply it to your pressure points.

Different scents can help your mind and body in different ways. Here are a few scents that help alleviate anxiety:

- Lavender. Lavender oil has been rated as potent and effective at relieving anxious feelings. Lavender has been used to combat anxiety for quite some time and even helps with insomnia. This makes it one of the most popular essential oil fragrances, and a great choice for women with PCOS! Lavender calms anxiety by influencing your limbic system, the part of your brain that controls your emotions.
- Sage. All of the benefits of sage—flavor, scent, and more—come solely from its leaves. Sage

essential oil has a spicy and strong aroma. Diffusing sage essential oil will clarify and stimulate your mind while eliminating your fatigue and balancing your mood. When you buy sage essential oil, double-check the label, because there is also a clary sage essential oil. Clary sage might also calm you down and alleviate anxiety symptoms, but it will have a different scent and different effect than sage essential oil.

- Rosemary. Rosemary essential oil is extracted from the plant's leaves and gives off a strong, woody fragrance. Research shows that the scent of rosemary oil improves brain functions and reduces your anxiety by decreasing the levels of your stress hormones.
- Lemon. Lemon essential oil is extracted from the plant's leaves and the lemon's rind, which gives the oil a strong citrus scent. Lemon is a popular scent because it is associated with freshness, cleanliness, and sunshine. Make sure you buy lemon essential oil, not lemongrass. Lemongrass essential oil is an oil that smells similar to lemon, but lemongrass does not relieve anxiety. If you buy lemongrass instead of lemon essential oil, you will not get the anti-anxiety benefits you need.

- Bergamot orange. Bergamot orange essential oil has a bright citrus scent that is calming and will uplift your mood.
- Neroli. While bergamot orange essential oil has a vibrant citrus scent, neroli essential oil has a floral scent with a hint of orange. The smell of neroli essential oil sends messages to the limbic system, which then influences the nervous system to slow your heart rate, which will lower your stress levels.
- Ylang-ylang. Ylang-ylang oil smells fruity and flowery, and studies show that the scent leads to heightened self-esteem, which is a positive side effect when it comes to trying to lower your stress. Self-esteem is also great for self-care, and something that a lot of women with PCOS lack, so ylang-ylang oil is a good one to try.
- Chamomile. Chamomile is a popular tea because sipping it calms your anxiety and soothes your stomach. Drinking chamomile tea at bedtime also helps you get a good night's sleep. Whether you drink chamomile tea or just want to use the oil, the scent will greatly benefit you. Chamomile has a sweet and fresh scent, but there is also a smoky base note that has a grounding effect on your moods, keeping your emotions balanced.

- Sweet basil. Sweet basil oil has a warm, crisp floral scent with a faint hint of licorice. Sweet basil has been used in Indian holistic practices as an antioxidant, anti-inflammatory, and more. Sweet basil has been found to have stress-relieving compounds like the ones found in diazepam, an anxiety medication. Except sweet basil oil is natural, so you do not have to take a pill or worry about any side effects.

Do not worry about the brand name of the essential oil, just carefully read the label. A quality essential oil brand will include the plant's Latin name on the label, along with the country of origin and the date of production. If a certain brand sounds good to you, research them more before buying. The brand's website should have information about safety tests they conducted and the standards they meet.

Picking the best essential oil for anxiety is a personal decision, as it depends on each individual's smell receptors. A fragrance might smell calming to you, but it might irritate someone else.

Anxiety is also very personal, so it might affect you in one way, and a certain smell might not be the best compliment for that feeling. After reading about the oils above, you might want to buy a sampler kit and test out different fragrances on your own.

Clear Mental Roadblocks

There are different ways you can clear mental roadblocks depending on what seems to be bothering you. Obviously being preoccupied with grief after losing a loved one is different than being upset over something that happened at work. Focusing on some ways you can clear the smaller mental roadblocks that challenge you every day will help you know how you can tackle the bigger problems when they come up.

Writing things down can help keep your mind clear. You can have a journal specifically for this purpose. Once you write something down, it is out of your mind. You might still want to think about it, but you should know that writing it down releases it. You do not have to write a journal entry if you would rather just write word association around a feeling that seems to be dominating your day.

You could also write a list of things that have bothered you. Or, to put a positive spin on it, you can write a list of positive things that happened to you each day. Doing this before bed is a good activity to clear your mind, relieve stress, and put you in a happy state of mind before drifting off to sleep.

You can do this activity first thing in the morning if you would rather start your day with a clean slate. Writing morning pages is a practice that many writers, artists, and creatives have done for years. They wake up and write their first thoughts, before checking email or having a conversation with someone else. This way they are distilling pure thoughts on the paper, and these thoughts are often joyful ones they can look back on at the end of the day, or anytime later when they need to be reminded of all they should be grateful for.

A fun way to clear mental roadblocks is to laugh. Listen to a stand-up comedian's set or read a funny book. Watch your favorite sitcom. Anything that lets your mind feel free enough to laugh will help reduce stress and take your mind off anything that is bothering you. Whenever the negative thoughts come back to you, you will be in a happier state of mind. They might not seem as serious or stressful since you took a step back from them.

Practicing mindfulness is a great way to clear mental roadblocks and relieve stress. Mindfulness challenges you to be present in each moment of your life. Instead of remembering the past or worrying about the future, you are only thinking about the present moment. Mindfulness does not mean you have to sit quietly and meditate, though that can be helpful, and is definitely a form of self-care. Mindfulness can actually be social, because if you are focusing on each moment then you are sure to enjoy the people you are with to the fullest.

Mindfulness engages all of your senses so you always feel present. You are seeing everything around you. You are smelling any scents and identifying where they come from. You are noticing things of beauty. You are breathing deeply and feeling the air in your lungs. You are grateful to be alive and to be feeling everything in this moment.

When you are practicing mindfulness, you are not judging anything. You are not thinking, "That smells bad. Someone cannot cook; they burned their lunch." You are simply noticing everything and allowing the thoughts to float on by after you think them. If you notice yourself lingering on one thought, let it go and move on to something else. The act of being mindful for a few minutes should almost feel like you are sweeping thoughts from your mind so you are left with a clear surface.

If you take deep breaths while practicing mindfulness, you will feel stress melt away from your body. Close your eyes and work on relaxing your body from your head to your toes. Allow yourself to be totally relaxed while making time for mindful moments.

You do not have to be sitting down or lying down to have a mindful moment; this can happen while you walk or exercise too. It is not a strict practice that demands a lot of your body, it is something that can be done in conjunction with other activities. It should not be a passive practice, though. You should be focusing on your thoughts first and foremost.

If you feel like you want to be mindful or practice meditation but are struggling to do it on your own, consider doing some research into the field. Learning more about mindfulness will help you realize how easy it is to practice no matter where you are or what you are doing. There are also guided meditation and mindfulness apps that you can download and use to help you practice this method of stress management.

Overcome Challenges

Mindfulness will help you overcome a lot of challenges, but you should also have a bottom line as a go-getter. It can be hard to be motivated when you are suffering from PCOS, but procrastinating only makes things worse. This does not mean you have to accomplish ten major projects every day—you can rank your priorities and focus on what is most important. You can break the larger tasks into smaller duties so you can feel proud of the progress you are making bit by bit.

When you procrastinate, you become unmotivated and get left behind. You have to scramble to catch up, but you are so used to letting things go that it is harder to get back to your usual work ethic and level of productivity. Procrastination might feel good in the moment—who would not rather take a nap than take out the trash? But putting off tasks will only stress you out more. You will find yourself constantly thinking about them until you do them, so just get them out of the way as soon as you can. You will eliminate stress and be able to sleep better at night.

Time management will help you both with your To-Do list and overcoming challenges in general. You do not need to set aside two hours to clean your house, because that can be exhausting and boring. If you lose steam halfway through, you are less likely to come back to the task, and instead go back to procrastinating on completing it. Instead, break it into manageable portions and give yourself a set time to complete each part. Set a timer for twenty minutes and clean your kitchen. When the timer goes off, take a five-minute break to step outside for some fresh air or read a few pages of your book. Then come back and set your timer for another twenty minutes, and tackle your next task.

Instead of burning out on a task by working until it is done, this method gives you a set time to finish things. You might find that twenty minutes is too long for your tasks, and you can either change the time limit or enjoy a few more minutes of relaxation. Remember, time management is a way to practice self-care, so you should not press yourself or else you will feel stressed again.

Avoid Endocrine Disruptors

Endocrine disruptors are chemicals that cause problems in your endocrine system. Your endocrine system is what produces and balances all of your hormones, so if you have PCOS then you already know how fragile this system can be. If you can avoid anything that will disrupt your natural hormones, whether the production of them or the balance of them, you definitely should.

Endocrine disruptors are often found in everyday items like beauty and hygiene products, fragrances, food and its packaging, things made of plastic, and tap water. Research has found that endocrine disruptors have been linked to severe complications such as cancer, thyroid disease, birth defects, and other developmental disorders. Babies and children are at the most risk for adverse effects, but since women with PCOS already have hormone issues, you want to be aware of what endocrine disruptors you might be encountering every day.

There are a few common endocrine disruptors you will likely encounter daily. They include:

- Bisphenol A, or BPA, which is used to make plastic containers and bottles. It can be found in the lining of canned goods and other food-packaging materials. It is even found in the thermal paper of cash register receipts. Research has found that BPA can cause breast and other cancers, reproductive and fertility issues, and obesity—all things that women with PCOS are especially susceptible to.
- Phthalates are chemicals found in fragrances, plastic, and plastic toys. Research has found that exposure to phthalates can cause miscarriages and gestational diabetes. You can avoid this chemical by staying away from plastic and fragrances. Remember that fragrances are not just perfumes and deodorants—many other

items contain fragrances, like wipes, diapers, and even garbage bags.
- Flame retardants are pretty much everywhere: in mattresses, cushions, furniture, insulation, and electronics. Flame retardant chemicals have been found to cause hormone disruption, some types of cancer, and attention deficits in children. The United States has phased out many of the most toxic flame retardant chemicals, but they were replaced with alternatives that might not be much healthier.

You can avoid these endocrine disruptors by:
- Eating more plants. Endocrine disruptors are found in meat and food packaging, so eating as much fresh food as you can will help.
- Filter your water. Your tap water might have endocrine disruptors in it, but if you attach a filter to your faucet, you can still drink it. Some glass water pitchers also have lids fitted with filters, so you could keep cold water in your refrigerator with one of these pitchers. Do not buy bottled water instead of drinking from the tap, because plastic bottles also contain endocrine disruptors.
- Cook using stainless steel or cast iron. The non-stick coating on many of your pots and pans is

made from perfluorinated chemicals, which contain endocrine disruptors.
- Stop using plastic. This includes buying food and drinks packaged in plastic, using plastic wrap to save your leftovers, and buying plastic toys and jewelry. Not only will this help you avoid endocrine disruptors, but you will also help save the environment! Cans may be better for the environment, but even canned goods contain endocrine disruptors, so eat fresh food as much as possible.
- Always read the labels. Beauty and hygiene products have a lot of endocrine disruptors in them, so look for products with natural ingredients. You can even make your own perfumes and deodorants from baking soda and natural oils.

In addition to taking these steps to eliminate endocrine disruptors from your daily life, you can also stay safe by frequently washing your hands, and vacuuming your house often. When you clean, use natural cleaning solutions instead of harsh chemicals. Making your own cleaning solutions with vinegar and baking soda is not only healthier and better for the environment, but it will also save you money because those products can be bought in bulk at affordable prices.

Chapter 5:

Your PCOS Diet

One common thread you have probably been noticing throughout learning about all aspects of PCOS is that having a healthy diet that can help you manage your symptoms. Women diagnosed with PCOS usually have higher than average insulin levels. Since insulin helps the cells in your body turn sugar into energy, if it is not being regulated properly, you will have some diet and weight problems.

A lot of women with PCOS are insulin resistant, which means you are not able to use the insulin you do produce effectively, so you gain weight or are unable to lose the weight you have. Since your body cannot use the insulin it produces, it constantly sends signals to your brain that you need more, so you are often craving sugar that you do not need.

A diet high in refined carbohydrates, like sugar or starchy foods, can make insulin resistance more difficult to control. This makes it harder for you to lose weight. But if you follow a diet approved for PCOS, you will be more likely to be healthier, keep your insulin levels balanced, and be able to stay at an ideal weight.

What to Add to or Remove From Your Diet

Certain foods help manage PCOS symptoms by providing you with healthy fats and nutrients you need to eat a balanced diet yet still feel satisfied. There are also foods that are bad for you and might trigger your symptoms so they flare up and cause more harm.

Foods to Add

It is important to eat natural and unprocessed foods to manage your PCOS symptoms. You will also want to add a lot of fiber and protein.

High-Fiber Foods

Fiber is any type of carbohydrate that your body does not digest. High-fiber foods help lower insulin resistance by slowing down your digestion and reducing the impact of sugar on your body's overall health. Fiber is incredibly important because it passes through your stomach without being digested and ends up in your colon, where it feeds good bacteria, leading to various health benefits like weight loss and lower blood sugar levels. It is recommended that you eat fourteen grams of fiber for every one thousand calories you eat daily, which means that most women should eat at least twenty-four grams of fiber a day.

Benefits of fiber include:

- Reduced cholesterol. Since your body does not digest fiber, it being present in your digestive tract can prevent your body from absorbing cholesterol, which is a very good thing!
- Maintaining an ideal weight. High-fiber foods are usually lower in calories, like vegetables and fruits. Fiber also slows digestion so you feel fuller for longer, meaning you will not eat as much or snack as often.
- Controlling blood sugar. Since it takes your body a long time to break down fiber, you can maintain more evenly balanced blood sugar levels.
- Lowering the risks of gastrointestinal cancer. Some fibers have antioxidant properties that help prevent certain types of cancer, including colon cancer.

After learning about all the benefits, you are probably eager to add fiber to your diet. Make sure you increase your fiber intake gradually, so you do not throw your digestive system off track. Since fiber can cause constipation, you do not want to clog your intestines. High-fiber foods include:

- cruciferous vegetables, such as broccoli, cauliflower, and Brussels sprouts
- fruits like apples, pears, strawberries, raspberries, and bananas
- lettuce, kale, and arugula
- green and red peppers
- avocados
- carrots
- beets
- artichokes
- beans, chickpeas, edamame, and lentils
- oats, popcorn, almonds, and chia seeds
- sweet potatoes, squash, and pumpkin

Lean Protein

Some sources of protein might include more fat and calories than you want to add to your diet, but lean proteins will keep you at your caloric intake goal. Lean protein does not add fiber to your diet, but these options are very filling, so they are good choices for meals with a high-fiber side to keep your energy levels high and prevent you from snacking.

Protein helps build and maintain muscle and also helps manage your weight. Women should eat at least fifty grams of lean protein a day, though women diagnosed with PCOS might benefit from eating more. Examples of lean protein include:

- fish, such as haddock, flounder, cod, halibut, pollock, tilapia, and orange roughy
- plain, non-fat Greek yogurt (you can add your own fruit for flavor)
- lentils, beans, and peas
- skinless white-meat poultry, such as breasts, tenderloins, and wings of chickens and turkeys
- lean beef, or cuts labels 'round' or 'loin'
- pork loin
- frozen, unbreaded shrimp
- bison
- tofu
- low-fat cottage cheese
- low-fat milk
- egg whites

Anti-Inflammatory Foods

Chronic inflammation can lead to weight gain, so it is important that women with PCOS avoid inflammatory foods. Some food that can fight inflammation include:

- strawberries, blueberries, raspberries, and blackberries
- fish like salmon, herring, sardines, anchovies, and mackerel
- bell peppers and chili peppers

- kale
- spinach
- mushrooms
- broccoli
- tomatoes
- avocado
- grapes
- cherries
- almonds and walnuts
- green tea
- turmeric
- extra virgin oil olive
- dark chocolate

You probably noticed that a lot of these foods are repeated across lists, especially the high-fiber and anti-inflammatory foods. Hopefully you will be able to find easy ways to incorporate these foods to your diet since they will provide so many benefits for your health.

Foods to Remove

You will want to avoid some foods because they are unhealthy, will cause your hormones to be disrupted, or cause your PCOS symptoms to flare. You want to avoid refined carbohydrates, sugar, and inflammatory foods.

Refined Carbohydrates

Refined carbohydrates often cause inflammation and worsen your insulin resistance, so you should avoid eating them as much as possible. Refined carbohydrates include:

- white bread, or anything made with white flour
- muffins, breakfast pastries, and sugary desserts
- pasta noodles made with white or wheat flour
- sugary sodas and juice
- white rice
- white potatoes
- instant oatmeal
- corn or potato chips

Sugar

A lot of the sugary items will be self-explanatory—and a lot were already seen on the refined carbohydrates list. Make sure you check the ingredients list before you eat a food, and if it lists sugar, sucrose, dextrose, or high fructose corn syrup towards the beginning of the list, do not eat it. Stay away from:

- cakes, cookies, and sugary desserts
- sweetened cereal
- yogurt with additional sugar
- sweetened instant oatmeal
- ice cream

- sweetened smoothies
- fruit juice
- sodas
- candy

Inflammatory Foods

You know you want to eat anti-inflammatory foods, but what foods are inflammatory? They include:

- food made with sugar or high fructose corn syrup
- artificial trans fats, like that found in margarine, fried food, fast food, processed food, and vegetable shortening
- vegetable and seed oils, like soybean, sunflower, olive, and coconut
- refined carbohydrates, as detailed above
- processed meat
- excessive alcohol

Three Diets That May Help People with PCOS

From the lists of foods to add and avoid above, and the recipes that will be shared later, you can cobble together a healthy diet to help manage your PCOS symptoms. However, there are three general diets that have helped women with PCOS manage their weight and stay healthy for years. You can use these as guidelines as you create your own diet, or you can pick one that sounds good and follow it more strictly.

Anti-Inflammatory Diet

An anti-inflammatory diet can help with weight loss and prevent heart attacks. It is typically full of foods like fatty fish, fresh greens, extra virgin olive oil, and berries. You can create your own anti-inflammatory diet from the list of anti-inflammatory foods given above, or you can follow a set anti-inflammatory diet, like the Mediterranean diet. You can substitute any food that does not strike your fancy with something similar that better suits your taste, just make sure you stick with the general food type and serving size for the best benefits.

An anti-inflammatory diet is full of plant foods and low in animal foods, but it is recommended that you eat fish and seafood at least twice a week. This diet works best if you use whole, single-ingredient foods so you know what you are eating is pure and healthy.

Foods to Eat

Make sure you eat plenty of:

- Vegetables like tomatoes, cucumbers, broccoli, Brussels sprouts, kale, cauliflower, spinach, onions, and carrots
- Fruits like apples, oranges, pears, melons, bananas, peaches, strawberries, dates, figs, and grapes
- Nuts and seeds like pumpkin seeds, almonds, macadamia nuts, hazelnuts, walnuts, cashews, and sunflower seeds
- Legumes like peas, chickpeas, beans, lentils, and peanuts
- Tubers like turnips, potatoes, sweet potatoes, and yams
- Whole grains like whole oats, whole wheat, rye, barley, brown rice, corn, whole wheat, and pasta
- Fish and seafood like salmon, clams, crab, sardines, tuna, mackerel, trout, shrimp, oysters, and mussels
- Poultry like chicken, turkey, and duck
- Eggs from chickens, ducks, and quail
- Dairy like cheese, yogurt, and Greek yogurt

- Herbs and spices to add flavor, like garlic, pepper, rosemary, sage, basil, mint, nutmeg, and cinnamon
- Healthy Fats like olives, extra virgin olive oil, avocados, and avocado oil.

You should drink mostly water on this diet, but red wine has antioxidant properties, as long as you do not drink more than one glass a day. You can also drink coffee and tea, as long as you do not add too much cream and sugar.

Snack Options

The anti-inflammatory diet is made so the meals should be filling enough on their own, but if you get hungry throughout the day, choose from these healthy snack options:

- a piece of fruit
- apple slices with almond butter
- a handful of nuts
- carrots
- berries or grapes
- Greek yogurt
- leftovers from last night's anti-inflammatory dinner.

Sample Meal Plan

A sample meal plan for the week will give you an idea about how you can implement the foods listed above into a well-rounded meal. The dinner ideas typically make enough for two to four servings, so you can pack them as leftovers for lunches later in the week.

Day One

Breakfast: Greek yogurt topped with your choice of berries and whole oats

Lunch: Sandwich on whole-grain bread with a side of raw vegetables

Dinner: Tuna salad with a light topping of olive oil and a piece of fruit

Day Two

Breakfast: Oatmeal topped with raisins or a chopped banana

Lunch: Tuna salad left over from last night

Dinner: Leafy green salad topped with tomatoes, feta cheese and olives

Day Three

Breakfast: Omelet with diced tomatoes and onions with a piece of fruit on the side

Lunch: Sandwich made with cheese and fresh vegetables on whole-grain bread

Dinner: Mediterranean lasagna made with whole-grain pasta

Day Four

Breakfast: Yogurt parfait layered with sliced fruits and nuts

Lunch: Lasagna leftover from last night

Dinner: Salmon with brown rice and vegetables

Day Five

Breakfast: Eggs and vegetables mixed with olive oil

Lunch: Greek yogurt topped with your choice of berries, nuts, and oats

Dinner: Grilled lamb or steak with a leafy green side salad and baked potato

Day Six

Breakfast: Oatmeal mixed with raisins and nuts with an apple on the side

Lunch: Sandwich made from whole-grain bread with vegetables

Dinner: Mediterranean pizza with a whole-wheat crust, topped with feta cheese, olives, and other vegetables as suit your taste

Day Seven

Breakfast: Omelet mixed with veggies

Lunch: Pizza left over from last night

Dinner: Grilled chicken with a side of vegetables and a potato with a piece of fruit.

Low Glycemic Index Diet

The glycemic index is a health tool that is used to help you improve your blood sugar management. A food's glycemic index is based on its nutrient composition, the cooking method, its ripeness, and the amount of processing it goes through. The glycemic index helps you increase your awareness of what you eat while also decreasing your blood sugar levels, reducing your cholesterol and improving your chances of losing weight.

Your body digests food with lower glycemic indexes slowly, so your insulin levels will not rise as quickly as they do when you eat other foods, like carbs. To follow a low glycemic index diet you will be eating a lot of nuts, whole grains, fruits, starchy vegetables, and low-carbohydrate foods.

Foods to Eat

You do not have to count calories or track your fat, protein, or carbs on the low glycemic index diet, instead, you will just be making healthier choices of foods with low glycemic indexes. You can eat:

- Bread that is whole grain, multigrain, sourdough, or rye
- Breakfast cereals like bran flakes or those made from steel-cut oats
- Fruit like kiwi, apricots, apples, peaches, strawberries, plums, and pears
- Vegetables like carrots, cauliflower, broccoli, zucchini, and celery
- Starchy vegetables like sweet potatoes, yams, winter squash, and corn
- Legumes like lentils, baked beans, butter beans, chickpeas, and kidney beans
- Pasta, vermicelli noodles, and rice noodles
- Basmati rice, brown rice, and long grain rice
- Barley, quinoa, couscous, and semolina

- Milk, coconut milk, soy milk, almond milk, cheese, and yogurt
- Fish like tuna, salmon, trout, and sardines
- Other meat like chicken, lamb, beef, and pork
- Nuts like macadamia nuts, almonds, cashews, walnuts, and pistachios
- Fats and oils like butter, olive oil, and avocado oil
- Herbs and spices like salt, pepper, garlic, basil, and dill

Snack Options

If you get hungry between meals, these snacks have low glycemic indexes:

- a handful of raw unsalted nuts
- a cup of berries or grapes served with a few cubes of cheese
- a piece of fruit with a nut butter of your choice
- carrot sticks dipped in hummus
- Greek yogurt topped with sliced almonds
- a hard-boiled egg
- leftovers from last night's low glycemic index meal.

Sample Meal Plan

A sample meal plan for the week will give you an idea about how you can implement the foods listed above into a well-rounded meal. The dinner ideas typically make enough for two to four servings, so you can pack them as leftovers for lunches later in the week.

Day One

Breakfast: oatmeal made from rolled oats with milk, pumpkin seeds, and a fresh, chopped fruit from the low glycemic index list

Lunch: chicken sandwich on whole-grain bread with a salad on the side

Dinner: beef and vegetable stir-fry served on long grain rice

Day Two

Breakfast: whole-grain toast topped with tomato, avocado, and smoked salmon

Lunch: minestrone soup with a slice of whole-grain bread on the side

Dinner: grilled fish with a side of broccoli and green beans

Day Three

Breakfast: omelet made with mushrooms, tomato, spinach, and cheese

Lunch: salmon and quinoa with a salad on the side

Dinner: homemade pizza made with a whole-wheat crust

Day Four

Breakfast: smoothie made with milk, Greek yogurt, your choice of berries, and cinnamon to taste

Lunch: chicken pasta salad made using whole-wheat pasta

Dinner: beef burger patties topped with vegetables, served on whole-wheat buns

Day Five

Breakfast: quinoa mixed with apple and cinnamon

Lunch: tuna sandwich on whole-wheat bread

Dinner: chicken and chickpea curry served with basmati rice

Day Six

Breakfast: eggs with tomatoes served on whole-grain toast

Lunch: whole-grain wrap made with egg and lettuce

Dinner: grilled lamb chops with a side of greens and mashed sweet potato

Day Seven

Breakfast: pancakes made from buckwheat and served with your choice of berries

Lunch: brown rice and tuna

Dinner: beef meatballs served with vegetables on top of brown rice

Dietary Approaches to Stop Hypertension (DASH) Diet

The Dietary Approaches to Stop Hypertension (DASH) diet is often prescribed to reduce the risk of heart disease, but it also works well to manage PCOS symptoms. The DASH diet excludes foods that are high in sugar and saturated fats. Instead, you will eat a lot of fruits, vegetables, fish, and poultry.

Foods to Eat

The DASH diet does not list specific foods to eat, but instead is strict about the serving size you eat from each food group.

Eat six to eight servings of grains every day, such as whole-wheat and whole-grain bread, whole-grain breakfast cereals, oatmeal, brown rice, and quinoa.

Eat four to five servings of vegetables every day. The DASH diet has no restrictions on what vegetables you can eat.

Eat four to five servings of fruit every day. The DASH diet makes room for a lot of fruit, and typically asks that you eat at least one a day as a snack. These fruits include peaches, berries, apples, pears, and tropical fruits like mango and pineapple.

Eat two to three servings of dairy products every day. The dairy you consume on the DASH diet should be low fat, like skim milk, low-fat yogurt, and low-fat cheese.

Eat less than six servings of lean meat every day. This includes eggs, lean chicken, and fish, but you can eat red meat once or twice a week.

Eat four to five servings of nuts, legumes, and seeds every week. These servings can be almonds, hazelnuts, peanuts, walnuts, lentils, split peas, kidney beans, sunflower seeds, and flaxseed. Nut butters are also included in this category.

Eat two to three servings of fats and oils every day. The DASH diet prioritizes vegetable oils over anything else. Vegetable oils include canola oil, olive oil, corn oil, margarine, low-fat mayonnaise, and light salad dressing.

Eat five or fewer servings of candy and sweet treats every week. This includes any candy, adding table sugar to any drinks or food, drinking soda, using jelly or jam, or using artificial sweeteners like agave nectar.

Snack Options

The DASH diet plans meals to fill you eat in each sitting, but if you get hungry during the day you can choose from healthy snacks like:

- almonds
- an apple
- a banana
- an orange
- a cup of low-fat yogurt
- canned peaches, pears, or pineapple
- fruit salad
- crackers and cottage cheese
- homemade yogurt parfait layered with berries

Sample Meal Plan

Since the DASH diet is strict about the serving size you eat from each food group, this meal plan is more detailed than that of the previous two diets.

Day One

Breakfast: one cup of oatmeal mixed with one cup of skim milk, topped with half a cup of blueberries with half a cup of fresh orange juice to drink

Lunch: three ounces of canned tuna mixed with one tablespoon of light mayonnaise to make a sandwich using two slices of whole-grain bread, with one and a half cups of green salad on the side

Dinner: three ounces of lean chicken breast cooked in one teaspoon of vegetable oil, stir-fried with half a cup of broccoli and half a cup of carrots, served over one cup of brown rice

Day Two

Breakfast: two slices of whole-wheat toast topped with one teaspoon of margarine and one tablespoon of jelly or jam, with half a cup of fresh orange juice to drink and one medium apple as a side

Lunch: three ounces of lean chicken breast tossed with two cups of green salad, tossed with one and a half ounces of low-fat cheese and one cup of brown rice on the side

Dinner: three ounces of salmon cooked in one teaspoon of vegetable oil, served with one cup of boiled potatoes and one and a half cups of other boiled vegetables

Day Three

Breakfast: one cup of oatmeal mixed with one cup of skim milk and half a cup of blueberries with half a cup of fresh orange juice to drink

Lunch: sandwich made from two slices of whole-wheat bread, three ounces of lean turkey, one and a half ounces of low-fat cheese, served with half a cup of green salad topped with half a cup of cherry tomatoes

Dinner: six ounces of cod fillet served with one cup of mashed potatoes, half a cup of green peas, and half a cup of broccoli

Day Four

Breakfast: one cup of oatmeal mixed with one cup of skim milk and topped with half a cup of raspberries with half a cup of fresh orange juice to drink

Lunch: two cups of green salad topped with four and a half ounces of grilled tuna, one hard-boiled egg, half a cup of cherry tomatoes, and two tablespoons of low-fat dressing

Dinner: three ounces of pork fillet served with one cup of mixed vegetables and one cup of brown rice.

Day Five

Breakfast: two hard-boiled eggs, two slices of turkey bacon, half a cup of cherry tomatoes, half a cup of baked beans, two slices of whole-wheat toast, and half a cup of orange juice to drink

Lunch: sandwich made from two slices of whole-wheat toast, topped with one tablespoon of low-fat mayonnaise and one and a half ounces of low-fat cheese, with a side salad made from half a cup of salad greens mixed with half a cup of cherry tomatoes

Dinner: one cup of spaghetti and four ounces of minced turkey-shaped into meatballs with half a cup of green peas on the side

Day Six

Breakfast: two slices of whole-wheat toast topped with two tablespoons of peanut butter, one medium banana cut into slices, with two tablespoons of mixed seeds sprinkled on top, and half a cup of fresh orange juice to drink

Lunch: three ounces of grilled chicken and one cup of roasted vegetables, served over one cup of couscous.

Dinner: three ounces of pork steak and one cup of ratatouille served with one cup of brown rice, half a cup of lentils, and one and a half ounces of low-fat cheese

Day Seven

Breakfast: one cup of oatmeal mixed with one cup of skim milk and topped with half a cup of blueberries with half a cup of fresh orange juice to drink

Lunch: chicken salad made from three ounces of lean chicken breast mixed with one tablespoon of mayonnaise, served with two cups of green salad topped with half a cup of cherry tomatoes and half a tablespoon of seeds, with four whole-grain crackers on the side

Dinner: three ounces of roast beef served with one cup of boiled potatoes, half a cup of broccoli, and half a cup of green peas.

Nutrients to Increase

In addition to balancing your diet with a lot of healthy foods, you might want to increase other nutrients that might not

Vitamin D and Calcium

Women who take metformin, which is a medication that can be used to treat PCOS symptoms, added supplements of vitamin D and calcium to their diets and saw improvements in their body mass index (BMI), regulations in their menstrual cycles, and a decrease in other PCOS other symptoms. If you are taking metformin, ask your doctor about adding in vitamin D and calcium supplements. The study added one thousand milligrams of daily calcium to the women's diets, and one hundred thousand international units (IU) of vitamin D a month.

If you do not want to take any supplements, you can make sure you are eating plenty of foods with vitamin D and calcium, such as:

- oily fish like salmon, sardines, mackerel, and herring
- leafy greens like collard greens, spinach, and kale
- fortified foods like bread spreads and breakfast cereals
- red meat
- liver
- seeds
- cheese
- yogurt
- rhubarb
- beans and lentils

- almonds
- whey protein
- egg yolks
- edamame
- tofu
- milk and soy milk
- figs

You can also get vitamin D naturally by being outside in the sunlight.

Iron

Women with PCOS often experience heavy bleeding during their menstrual cycles. This loss of blood can lead to an iron deficiency or anemia. If your doctor diagnosed you with anemia or an iron deficiency, come up with a plan together for how you can safely increase your iron intake. Your doctor might recommend adding iron-rich foods to your diet, including:

- red meat, poultry, and pork
- liver and organ meats
- seafood and shellfish
- turkey
- tofu
- dark green leafy vegetables like spinach
- broccoli
- dried fruit like raisins and apricots

- iron-fortified cereals, pastas, and breads
- beans, peas, seeds, and legumes
- dark chocolate

Magnesium

Women with PCOS typically have symptoms of insulin resistance and metabolic syndrome, which are risk factors that increase your risk for heart disease, diabetes, and strokes. Research indicates that a dietary supplement of magnesium can improve insulin sensitivity, which can potentially keep you from developing type 2 diabetes. If you do not want to take a magnesium supplement, you can eat these foods that are rich in magnesium:

- avocados
- tofu
- nuts like almonds, cashews, and Brazil nuts
- legumes like lentils, chickpeas, beans, peas, and soybeans
- leafy greens like kale, spinach, collard greens, mustard greens, and turnip greens
- whole grains like quinoa, buckwheat, oats, and barley
- seeds like flaxseed, pumpkin seeds, and chia seeds
- fatty fish like salmon, halibut, and mackerel
- bananas

- dark chocolate

Chromium

Consuming chromium lowers your fasting blood sugar and insulin levels to a degree that rivals the medication metformin. Chromium has also been linked to having positive effects on cholesterol levels, your risk of heart disease, managing Parkinson's disease, and lowering your risk of developing other health conditions. People also increase their chromium intake to help build muscle if they are weight training, or to trigger weight loss if they are trying to manage their weight.

If you are looking for a way to alleviate your PCOS symptoms without taking any medicine, consider adding foods rich in chromium to your diet:

- vegetables such as broccoli, green beans, and potatoes
- whole-grain breads and pastas
- beef and poultry
- fruits like apples, bananas, and grapes
- milk and dairy products like cheese and yogurt

Omega-3s

Fish oil has many health benefits, and research shows that omega-3 decreases androgen levels in women with

PCOS. Omega-3s are important protective parts of the cells in your body, especially in your eyes. Omega-3s can provide the calories necessary to give your body energy to get through the day. These healthy fats also have many benefits for your endocrine system, heart, blood vessels, immune system, and lungs. Instead of taking a supplement, get omega-3s naturally from:

- Cold-water fatty fish like salmon, sardines, anchovies, tuna, mackerel, oysters, and herring
- Nuts and seeds like walnuts, flaxseed, and chia seeds
- Plant oils like canola oil, flaxseed oil, and soybean oil
- Fortified foods like eggs, yogurt, milk, and juices
- Caviar
- Soybeans

Zinc

Zinc is a mineral that can boost your fertility as well as your immune system. Zinc is often found in cold medicines and throat lozenges. Consuming extra zinc can also help you manage your excessive hair growth. To get more zinc into your body, eat foods like:

- red meat, beef, pork, and lamb
- shellfish, crab, mussels, oysters, and shrimp
- legumes like lentils, chickpeas, and beans

- pumpkin seeds, squash seeds, and sesame seeds
- pine nuts, peanuts, almonds, and cashews
- dairy products like cheese and milk
- eggs
- whole grains like wheat, quinoa, oats, and rice
- potatoes, green beans, kale, and sweet potatoes

Other Tips

There are a lot of aspects to consider when you are managing your weight, but once you start to get your diet on track, all of these other pieces will fall into place.

Remember to be strategic with the calories you consume. The type of calories you eat and the time of day when you eat them can impact your glucose, insulin, androgen, and testosterone levels. Eating most of your calories at breakfast will improve your insulin and glucose levels, while eating your largest meal at dinner will not help you balance your hormones. A good way to plan your meals is to picture a pyramid, with breakfast at the base, being your largest meal with the most calories. Lunch is in the middle of the pyramid, having a moderate amount of calories. Dinner is the peak of the pyramid, and you should not consume too many calories at this meal. Eating less before bed will also help you get to sleep faster and sleep better throughout the night.

Even considering how your calorie intake will decrease throughout the day, you want to make sure you are eating healthy snacks regularly enough to keep your insulin levels stable. Women with PCOS usually find that the best schedule is to eat your three major meals at set times, but have a snack on hand to eat between each meal.

Practice mindful eating by being aware of how much you eat and drink. Note what times you seem hungriest or thirstiest, and what times you seem to have baseless cravings. Acknowledge the difference between your body actually feeling hungry and your mind telling your body that it is hungry. Also be conscious of what foods and drinks you choose to consume and when. If you know you get a sugar craving after work, you can shift your meal plan or calorie intake to accommodate that craving in a healthy way.

Fertility friendly eating tips for PCOS include eating a bigger breakfast and a smaller dinner, like the pyramid of calorie intake previously described. Eat more protein, greens, and complex carbohydrates like whole grains and beans. Make sure you are eating enough of these during your mealtime to cut down on your snacking in between meals.

Long-term calorie restriction will slow down your metabolism in time and change how your hormones operate. This can keep you from losing weight in the future, so make sure you are always eating the recommended amount of calories for your weight and height. This should be something you go over with your doctor when you start working on a weight loss and diet plan.

Meal and Snack Suggestions

It can be hard to make good food choices if you let yourself get too hungry, or if you find recipes that call for ingredients you will never find in your local grocery store. These recipes include ideas for breakfast, lunch, dinner, and snacks, and are made with easy to find ingredients. Most of them are pretty easy to make, but you can always make some meals in bulk, and meal plan for a week or two at a time. Having meals already prepared in your refrigerator or freezer will take some stress off of you while ensuring you will be making good food choices.

Breakfast

The popular adage claims that breakfast is the most important meal of the day, but if you are suffering from PCOS symptoms, it might be hard to get up and go in the mornings. Eating might be the last thing on your mind, but these recipes will have your mouth-watering for the first meal of the day!

You do not have to have a full meal for breakfast. If you just want to get some energy, then you can have some protein, like hard-boiled eggs, Greek yogurt, or a smoothie made with protein powder. Nuts and nut butters have healthy fats that can give you a boost of energy, and oatmeal is a good choice because of the complex carbohydrates it contains.

Yogurt Parfait

Ingredients:

- one cup of Greek yogurt
- half a cup of fresh berries
- one-fourth cup of granola

The fun thing about parfaits is they can be as fancy or plain as you want them to be! Your half cup of berries can be half a cup of strawberries, or it can be half a cup of strawberries, blueberries, and blackberries mixed together. You can layer granola, yogurt, fruit, yogurt, and top it all off with more granola. Or you can just toss it all together and eat it before you get your day started.

Avocado Toast

You will need:

- half an avocado
- a piece of whole-wheat bread

Toast your whole-grain bread and slice the avocado on top. If you cannot find a good avocado at the store, you can buy premade guacamole and use that instead!

Oatmeal

Oatmeal sounds like a boring old breakfast, but there is a reason it is a classic meal! There are many different types of oatmeal you can choose from, as long as you do not choose an instant oatmeal. Instant oatmeal is not as healthy because it has added sugar and other substances you do not need in your diet.

Once you have your oatmeal, you can add a lot of flavor by stirring in vanilla almond milk or add healthy fats by stirring in a tablespoon of nut butter.

Breakfast Scramble

Using a lot of the key breakfast elements will help you make a tasty breakfast scramble. The ingredients here are merely suggestions because you add in any vegetables and cheeses you have on hand and whip up a delicious meal.

You will need:

- one egg
- diced bell peppers
- mushrooms
- spinach

- one-fourth of a cup of shredded cheese
- one teaspoon of olive oil
- salt and pepper to taste
- hot sauce (if you want to add a kick!)

For the best-tasting scramble, you will want to sauté your vegetables in olive oil to get them tender before you add the eggs. Scramble the egg in a bowl before you add it to the skillet, and keep scrambling it with your spatula as you add the cheese and let it all cook.

Tomato and Egg Sandwich

Ingredients:
- one piece of whole-grain bread
- one egg, lightly beaten
- one-fourth of a tomato, diced
- one-fourth cup of shredded cheese
- salt, pepper, and garlic to taste

Scramble egg in a skillet and add diced tomatoes into the mix. You can add cheese at this point to get it melted, or you can save it to top off your sandwich. Toast your bread and add the egg mixture on top like an open-faced sandwich. If you did not melt your cheese into the egg mixture, you can sprinkle it on top of your sandwich now. Enjoy it while it is still warm!

Lunch

Some people eat lunch at home and some people want a lunch that is easy to pack and take along with them to work. I made sure to compile a mix of recipes that will suit you whether you are eating in your own kitchen at home, or packing a meal to go.

Bean and Tofu Salad

This recipe makes four servings, so it might be something you make one day and then enjoy leftovers for lunch the next few days.

You will need:

- one pack of extra firm tofu
- one small can of sliced olives
- two cans of chickpeas (can substitute kidney beans to suit your taste)
- two tablespoons of olive oil
- one tablespoon of lemon juice

Press the tofu to remove as much moisture as possible. Cut it into cubes. Add all of the other ingredients together and toss them in a bowl. Chill the salad for a few hours before serving.

Mozzarella and Tomato Pitas

This recipe makes two servings, so you can make it one day and still have another serving for the next day's lunch. Be sure to heat up the pita before you eat it as a leftover though—it tastes best warm!

Ingredients:

- one whole-wheat pita bread
- one ripe tomato
- two slices of skim milk mozzarella cheese
- four tablespoons of olive oil
- salt, pepper, and garlic to taste

Cut the pita bread in half so you have two bread pockets. Warm them up slightly in the oven or microwave. Chop the tomato and mix it in a bowl with the mozzarella. Add salt, pepper, and garlic to suit your taste. Drizzle the ingredients with olive oil, and then fill the warm pitas with the mixture.

Tuna Melt

This recipe makes four servings, believe it or not! You might want to make this if you are preparing lunch for several people. You can make it with the intention of eating leftovers, but you might want to make it all and only broil the one serving you will be eating for lunch. The other servings can be ready for future lunches, and you can broil them at the time when you are going to eat them. Because of course tuna melts are best served warm and melty!

You will need:

- two English muffins
- six ounces of canned tuna, drained
- four slices of cheese
- one-third of a cup of light mayonnaise (can substitute plain yogurt if you prefer)
- four tomato slices
- one and a half tablespoons of sweet relish
- half a tablespoon of mustard (optional)

Mix the tuna, mayonnaise, sweet relish, and mustard, if you choose to add it. Cut both English muffins in half and spread the tuna mixture on all four halves. Top each one with a slice of tomato and a slice of cheese. Broil them for about five minutes until the cheese melts.

Chicken Caesar Salad

Ingredients:

- half a head of lettuce
- one cooked chicken breast
- three slices of cooked bacon
- one tomato
- half a cucumber
- two hard-boiled eggs

- two tablespoons of Caesar dressing

Rip up the leaves of lettuce and lay them in a salad bowl. Cut the chicken breast into strips or bite-sized pieces. Dice the tomatoes and cucumbers and cut the eggs into coins or smaller pieces. Combine all of the ingredients in the bowl and crumble the bacon on top. Add the Caesar dressing and toss the salad all together before diving in!

Peanut Butter Banana Sandwich

This sandwich is a quick and easy meal that is healthy and full of healthy fats.

You will need:

- two pieces of whole-wheat bread
- two tablespoons of peanut butter (or another nut butter)
- half of a banana

Spread one tablespoon of peanut butter on each slice of bread. You can put all of the butter on one side, but applying a bit to both slices is a pro tip that will keep the banana slices from sliding out of the bread! Once you have peanut butter on both pieces of bread, cut the banana into circles and space them out according to your taste. Place the other piece of bread on top of the banana slices and enjoy. And rest assured that your banana slices will stay stuck to the peanut butter while you eat!

Dinner

After a long day, you might not feel like cooking, but a healthy homemade meal is a great way to end your day! I tried to find some of the most flavorful recipes that do not take a lot of effort to make. Most recipes here make four to six servings, so you can either cook for your whole family, have friends over, or save the leftovers to have later in the week for lunch and dinner!

Chicken Stir-Fry

This recipe makes six servings, so it is a great option to make for a family dinner, or if you want to prepare several days' worth of meals in advance.

You will need:
- six chicken breasts cut into bite-sized pieces
- two large onions, diced
- two large bell peppers, diced
- one cup of broccoli
- one carrot, cut into half-moons
- two cloves of garlic, minced
- three tablespoons of low-sodium soy sauce
- one tablespoon of canola oil
- three cups of brown rice

- salt and pepper to taste

Cook the brown rice according to the package. While it cooks, heat the oil in a skillet and sauté the chicken pieces. Put the chicken aside and add the onion, garlic, and bell pepper to the skillet. Add the carrots and broccoli and sauté all of the vegetables together. Stir the chicken back into the skillet and add soy sauce, salt, and pepper to taste. Serve half a cup of brown rice topped with a scoop of the chicken stir fry.

Vegetable Soup

This recipe makes five servings, so you can divide it up into smaller portions and save it in the refrigerator or freezer to warm up on some of those cold nights where you are craving some warm comfort food but do not feel like cooking!

Ingredients:
- two medium celery stalks
- two medium carrots
- one medium onion
- four small potatoes
- one clove of garlic
- one cup of dry lentils
- two fourteen ounce cans of chicken broth
- one sixteen-ounce can of stewed tomatoes
- three cups of water

- two tablespoons of olive, canola, or vegetable oil

Dice the celery stalks, carrots, and onion. Cut the potatoes into spoon-sized pieces. Mince the garlic. Heat the oil in a large pot, then add the celery, carrots, and onion and cook them until they are tender. Add garlic, then the can of stewed tomatoes—with the liquid. Add the dry lentils, potatoes, chicken broth, and water. Bring the pot to a boil and then reduce to a simmer. Cover and let it cook for about fifty minutes, or until the lentils are tender.

Basil Salmon

This recipe makes four servings, so it is a great suggestion for a healthy family dinner. You can also pack the servings up and eat them later in the week.

Ingredients:

- four cuts to salmon, each weighing six to eight ounces
- one tablespoon of fresh cut basil, or one teaspoon of dried basil
- two tablespoons of olive oil
- two tablespoons of lemon juice

Mix the lemon juice, basil, and olive oil together to brush on all sides of the salmon steaks. Grill the salmon, or cook in a skillet until the fish flakes with a fork.

Sushi Rice

This recipe makes a large portion of sushi rice so you can eat it for many meals, or use it as a smaller side if you make chicken breasts or salmon for future dinners.

Ingredients:

- one and a fourth cup of brown rice
- one-fourth cup wild rice
- one-fourth cup lentils
- one-fourth cup quinoa
- three tablespoons ground flaxseed
- four cups of warm water

Add the brown rice, wild rice, quinoa, lentils, and flaxseed with the water in a large pot. Let it soak at room temperature for thirty minutes to four hours so the grains can hydrate. Cover the pot and bring to a boil, then reduce it to a simmer. Wait until the liquid has all boiled off, for about thirty minutes. Remove the pot from the heat and let it stand, with the cover on, for thirty more minutes. Uncover and let it cool for thirty minutes before serving.

Fried Chicken Tenders

Fried chicken usually is not a healthy food choice, but this recipe is a gluten-free and paleo option! It makes four servings of chicken, so it is a great family dinner, or you will have plenty of leftovers for future meals.

Ingredients:

- one pound of chicken tenderloins
- two eggs
- one and one-third cup of almond flour
- one teaspoon of garlic powder
- one teaspoon of paprika
- one teaspoon of salt
- one-fourth teaspoon of pepper
- one-third cup of coconut oil or avocado oil

Whisk the eggs together in a shallow bowl, and in a separate bowl combine the flour, garlic powder, paprika, and salt and pepper. Add the coconut or avocado oil to a skillet and heat it until it is sizzling hot. Coat the chicken tenderloin in the flour mixture, then dip it in the egg bowl. Put it back in the flour mixture and make sure it is completely coated. Put it in the skillet and let it cook until the coating is brown, then flip it over and cook it until the other side browns. Let the fried chicken tenderloins drain on a paper towel to remove excess oil. Work in batches until all of the chicken is fried.

Snacks

If you get hungry between meals, you do not have to reach for a processed snack to satisfy your craving. Try some of these fast, easy, and tasty snack recipes. I tried to include a mix of recipes that can be made spur-of-the-moment but easily enough to keep you from getting hangry, as well as some that can be made in advance and packed to take with you to work or any other outing where you might find yourself getting hungry!

Fruit Salad

This recipe makes four servings of fruit salad, so it is a good choice to make and have on hand for snack time later in the week.

You can make this fruit salad year-round using whatever fruits are in season at your grocery store! If you do not like any of the fruits included in the recipe, substitute your own in, but make sure you stick to the measurements given.

Ingredients:
- half a cup of strawberries
- half a cup of blueberries
- one cup of cubed seedless watermelon
- half of a cantaloupe, cubed
- half of a honeydew melon, cubed
- one banana, peeled and sliced

Wash all the berries, trim the tops of strawberries, and cut them in halves or quarters. Toss all of the fruits together in a big serving bowl and then scoop out four separate servings.

Fruit Smoothie

You will need:

- two cups of blueberries
- two cups of strawberries
- one cup of Greek yogurt
- one cup of milk
- two cups of ice
- one teaspoon of vanilla extract

Blend the blueberries and strawberries with the cup of Greek yogurt and the cup of milk. Add in the two cups of ice, and stir in a teaspoon of vanilla extract to enhance the flavor.

This recipe makes four servings of smoothie, so you can keep extra servings in the freezer. Simply get them out and thaw them in the refrigerator overnight before you plan to drink them.

Hummus

This recipe makes eight servings of hummus, so you can package it up into small containers to have on hand

and eat with vegetable sticks, crackers, or whole-wheat pita bread for an easy snack!

Ingredients:

- one can of chickpeas, drained and rinsed
- one large clove of garlic
- two-thirds cup of water
- half a teaspoon of salt
- three tablespoons of tahini
- two tablespoons of olive, canola, or vegetable oil
- two tablespoons of lemon juice

Blend all of the ingredients together until well mixed and creamy.

Ants on a Log

You will need:

- one stalk of celery
- one tablespoon of peanut butter or soy nut butter
- raisins

Wash the celery, trim both ends, and cut it into snack-sized sticks. Spread the sticks with your nut butter and top with raisins.

Chocolate Avocado Mousse

Just because you are eating healthily to manage your PCOS symptoms does not mean you cannot have a dessert and splurge a little! This dessert tastes rich and regal, but it is keto, low carb, sugar-free, and best of all, is not hard to make. It makes six servings, so make sure you do not eat it all at once!

Ingredients:

- two large ripe avocados
- one half cup of unsweetened cocoa powder
- one half cup of coconut cream
- one half cup of powdered sweetener
- one half teaspoon of vanilla extract
- one teaspoon of nutmeg
- a pinch of nutmeg, cinnamon, and sea salt, to taste

Are you ready for the steps to make this luscious dessert? Put all of the ingredients in a blender, and blend until smooth. That is it! Then divide it up into six serving bowls so you do not eat it all at once. Chill it until you are ready to serve.

Sample Meal Plan Menus

Sometimes it is easier to have set menus planned for a few days so you do not have to worry about what to eat. Here are three sample menus you can use on alternate days, or use as a template and fill in your own foods from the recipes previously shared. The meals are measured out to be the healthiest options for you, while also being incredibly filling meals. Even so, there are three small snacks included in the plan for days when you are feeling munchy!

Sample Menu #1

Breakfast: half a cup of cottage cheese, one peach, a whole-wheat English muffin toasted with two teaspoons of peanut butter, one cup of milk to drink

Morning snack: a cheese stick and half a cup of grapes

Lunch: tuna salad made from three ounces of tuna, half a cup of diced celery, and two teaspoons of light mayonnaise. Enjoy the tuna with whole-wheat crackers. Have a pear and a cup of milk along with it.

Afternoon snack: an apple with two teaspoons of peanut butter

Dinner: grill two ounces of steak tips, top half a baked potato with three-fourths cup of blue cheese, with a cup of sautéed spinach on the side

Evening snack: an apple with one-fourth cup of almonds

Sample Menu #2

Breakfast: make an omelet using two whole eggs, half an ounce of shredded cheese, one-fourth cup of peppers, one-fourth cup of onions, and two tablespoons of salsa. Have an orange and a cup of milk to drink.

Morning snack: one cup of celery dipped in three tablespoons of hummus

Lunch: make an English muffin pizza by spreading one-fourth cup of tomato sauce on top of a whole-wheat English muffin, top with two ounces of cheese, and toast it until the cheese is melted. Have fruit salad (see the snack recipe above!) as a side with a cup of milk to drink.

Afternoon snack: make your own trail mix by combining half a cup of lean or fiber cereal with two tablespoons of nuts and two tablespoons of dried fruit

Dinner: cook one cup of whole-wheat pasta and toss it with three ounces of baked chicken breasts, one cup of steamed broccoli, one tablespoon of olive oil, and top with two tablespoons of grated cheese.

Evening snack: blend one cup of milk with half of a frozen banana and one tablespoon of peanut butter to make a smoothie

Sample Menu #3

Breakfast: two hard-boiled eggs, half a cup of fruit, a cup of lean or fiber cereal in a cup of milk

Morning snack: one cup of carrots dipped in three tablespoons of hummus

Lunch: a salad made of two cups of spinach or lettuce mixed with one to two cups of other vegetables like onions, carrots, peppers, cucumbers, or tomatoes. Add half a cup of chickpeas and half a cup of feta cheese. Top with one tablespoon of oil and vinegar dressing. You can also have a small piece of whole-wheat pita bread on the side to really enjoy the Greek theme of the meal!

Afternoon snack: six ounces of plain yogurt mixed with half a cup of unsweetened berries and two tablespoons of slivered almonds

Dinner: four ounces of baked salmon, one cup of steamed broccoli, three-fourths cup of brown rice

Evening snack: one banana with two tablespoons of peanut butter, one cup of milk to drink

Flavor Tips

In addition to the delicious recipes listed above, consider making your own meals by taking items from the healthy foods lists shared from each diet. Add flavor by using some of these tips:

- Use fresh herbs for additional flavor—fresh mint can add a zing to coleslaw, canned beans, and fresh vegetables
- Roast vegetables with garlic, olive oil, and rosemary for a delicious side
- Instead of buying premade dressings, try making your own using olive oil, balsamic vinegar, and a teaspoon of Dijon mustard
- Use pesto sauce to flavor different meats, fish, or steamed salads.

Chapter 6:

Boosting Your Fertility

Sharon was diagnosed with PCOS at sixteen. At seventeen, she had to have one of her ovaries removed. While most cysts are harmless, some rupture and cause extreme pain. In Sharon's case, a large cyst had crushed her ovary. Sharon has gone through in vitro fertilization (IVF) and suffered six miscarriages. She says that the struggle to conceive has been the hardest part of having PCOS. She did not have trouble losing weight and maintaining a diet, but it still was not enough to enable her to carry a baby to term.

Lily was diagnosed with PCOS at seventeen, and has suffered four miscarriages in recent years. She is currently five weeks pregnant, but has not yet let herself feel hopeful. Her other miscarriages have happened near the six-week mark, so she is holding her breath until then. While the miscarriages feel almost unbearable to Lily, she wants to have a child and is researching other options that might help her in the future.

Erika has been able to conceive naturally, though she also suffers from miscarriages in the first trimester. Jeana, on the other hand, has never been able to get pregnant on her own. She is about to start her third round of IVF.

Many women have stories similar to Sharon and Lily, and some have experiences like Erika and Jeana. But the bottom line is that PCOS affects every woman in different ways, and everyone's lives are different. Some women want to have their own children, and some women just want to raise a child. Every option, emotion, and lifestyle choice is valid. If you want to have your own child, you can change your lifestyle and try to conceive naturally. If that does not work, you can try medications and assisted reproductive technologies. If you still are not having any success, you could consider adopting or fostering children.

But again, this decision is incredibly personal. If you only want to have biological children, do not let anyone guilt you about adopting a baby or becoming a foster parent. On the other hand, if you are ready to adopt instead of struggling with infertility, do not let anyone make you feel like you should have your own child first. This journey is yours and yours alone. While you hopefully have people you can talk to, they should be there to support you, not to tell you what choices to make.

If you feel like you need a third-party sounding board, talk to your doctor or gynecologist about therapists who have helped women struggling with infertility before. Talking to someone who knows what you are going through, yet who is not personally invested in your life, can help you keep everything in perspective.

Lifestyle Changes

Too often, the 'answer' doctors give to women with PCOS who are trying to conceive is "lose weight." That is a reasonable request if it is paired with other helpful information, but often doctors cannot give any solutions that work for most women. If you have been following the information in this book, then you are well on your way to living with a healthy weight and eating a balanced diet. Hopefully some of the solutions here have been working for you and let you feel like you at least have some control over a situation that is otherwise completely out of your hands.

The good news is, you can tell your doctor that you have been making all of the necessary lifestyle changes to manage PCOS and are ready to try and conceive. That shows your doctor that you are taking things seriously, doing your own research, and are willing to put in the work. If you can tell them that you have been eating a healthy diet and exercising for several months, you can move on to the next option in your journey to conceive.

Many of the lifestyle changes you have made to this point were made with the goal of regulating your menstrual cycles and improving your chances of ovulating. Losing weight can help reach these goals because if your body has less weight to maintain, it can balance your hormones more easily and reroute energy from fat to other body systems. Losing weight also helps your body regulate your insulin resistance, which can also help control your blood sugar and prevent gestational diabetes during your pregnancy.

If you are a smoker, quitting is a major lifestyle change that will improve your whole-body health. Giving up smoking will help you lose weight, especially if you trade the habit for healthy snacks or exercise. If you are having trouble quitting, ask your doctor for help. You might need to use a patch or gum if you cannot go cold turkey. If you feel like it is too hard, just remember that smoking can cause pregnancy loss, low birth weight, and premature delivery. Even if you easily got pregnant as a smoker, it could cause you to lose your baby over time, and increases the risk of sudden infant death syndrome (SIDS).

Cutting out alcohol is necessary, it should go without saying. Heavy alcohol binges are incredibly harmful to your own health and that of your baby, and drinking also decreases your chances of getting pregnant. Research goes back and forth on if you can have a drink here and there throughout your pregnancy, but it is best to avoid alcohol completely. You have done so much amazing work to get to this point, so you do not want to lose or harm your baby just for an alcoholic beverage.

Eliminating caffeine is also recommended to help you get pregnant. Drinking three to four cups of coffee, or sodas with that amount of caffeine in them, can decrease your possibility of conceiving. Research shows that drinking caffeine in the weeks leading up to your pregnancy can cause a miscarriage, so if you are actively trying to conceive, it is better to cut caffeine out completely, just to be safe.

As you undertake these lifestyle changes, start monitoring your cycles. If they are becoming more regular, this may help you pinpoint the month when you can start trying to conceive. As your menstruation regulates, you will also be able to find your window of ovulation. You can use ovulation tests to find out exact dates and increase your chance of getting pregnant naturally.

You do not have to wait until you are pregnant to start taking prenatal vitamins—you can start taking them when you are trying to conceive. Doctors actually recommend that you start taking prenatal vitamins three to six months before you hope to get pregnant, so adding in these vitamins might be one of your lifestyle changes. Prenatal vitamins contain folic acid, which can help prevent spinal deformities in your baby, but it also helps you throughout your pregnancy by helping your body produce and maintain new cells, prevent anemia, and even work against DNA changes that have been shown to lead to cancer.

Omega-3 fatty acid is another nutrient that your body and baby can benefit from. You have probably already started increasing your intake of this healthy fat, either by adding omega-3 rich foods to your diet or taking a supplement. Many prenatal vitamins also contain omega-3 fatty acids, so you can benefit from this during pregnancy.

Medication

If you are actively trying to conceive, your doctor might recommend you take medication to help the process. There are medications you can take to stimulate your body to release eggs so you can get pregnant. Your doctor might prescribe fertility drugs whether you are trying to conceive naturally or intend to use an assisted reproductive treatment.

Oral Medications

Doctors often prescribe medication to improve ovulation as a first approach to fertility treatment. These medications very often help women get pregnant naturally. If they do not help your situation, your doctor will then refer you to a fertility specialist for more focused approaches. Ovulation medications include:

- Metformin decreases insulin resistance, which can cause problems with ovulation. Taking metformin can help regulate your menstrual cycle while triggering your ovaries to produce eggs.
- Clomid is an estrogen-blocking drug that has been used to help women get pregnant for over forty years. Since it blocks your estrogen, Clomid tricks your body into thinking it needs

to make more of the hormone, which then triggers your ovaries to release eggs.
- Letrozole lowers your estrogen levels to increase your chance of ovulating. It is similar to Clomid, but has been proven to be more effective in women with PCOS, especially if they are overweight. Letrozole is also used to treat breast cancer in women who have gone through menopause.
- Dopamine agonists increase your dopamine levels and reduce the levels of a hormone called prolactin. Prolactin can prevent your ovaries from releasing an egg every month, so lowering that hormone while increasing your dopamine will help you ovulate regularly.
- Gonadotropins contain follicle-stimulating hormones that increase ovarian activity, including ovulation. This medication is also available as an injection or a nasal spray.

Injected Hormones

If the oral medications are not helping your ovulation, your doctor may recommend hormone injections. These are given as shots, some are just injected beneath the skin, while others must be injected into a muscle. Injections can be given on your stomach, buttocks, upper thigh, or upper arm. You will take your first injection the second or third day of your period, and take them continuously for seven to twelve days, depending on the dosage. You will give yourself these injections, so it is important to have a strong stomach and not be afraid of needles. Your skin and muscles might get sore at the injection site, but otherwise you should not experience negative side effects.

Some of the hormone injections available are:

- Human chorionic gonadotropin (hCG), which is usually used in conjunction with oral fertility drugs to trigger ovulation. Injections of hCG must be administered at a certain time in your menstrual cycle for maximum efficacy. Your doctor will be able to tell you when based on blood tests and ultrasounds. This hormone is actually found in the placenta during pregnancy, so it is safe and natural.
- Follicle-stimulating hormones (FSH) to trigger egg growth in your ovaries. Because FSH injections can be associated with a high risk of multiple pregnancy, triplets or more, some clinics prefer to prescribe other injections.
- Human menopausal gonadotropin (hMG) that includes follicle-stimulating hormones and luteinizing hormones. This injection includes both FSH and luteinizing hormone (LH) and will stimulate the ovaries to produce multiple eggs during one cycle. Injections of hMG are

usually given every day for seven to twelve days during the first half of your menstrual cycle.

Because IVF is so effective, many doctors and fertility clinics are phasing out injected hormones. Injected hormones have a ninety perfect success rate of helping a woman with PCOS ovulate regularly, but only a twenty percent success rate of natural pregnancy. They will still start you with oral medication to improve your fertility, but if those medicines do not help you get pregnant naturally, they often skip injectables completely and opt to start the IVF process.

Assisted Reproductive Technologies

If you have tried oral medications or injected hormones and still are not able to get pregnant naturally, your doctor might refer you to a fertility specialist who can help you take things to the next level. While you consider assisted reproductive technologies, you will most likely continue taking your medications or injections, because they will still help your body ovulate and be more receptive to conception.

You might want to consider starting fertility treatments right as you begin taking medications if you are in your late thirties. Since you are older, you might not want to take time to get your PCOS symptoms under control before working to get pregnant.

Keep in mind that fertility treatments do not help manage your PCOS symptoms in any way. While the medications and injections might help balance your hormones, fertility treatments themselves will only help you get pregnant, not address anything at the root level. Therefore, fertility treatments should not be seen as a solution for your PCOS struggle. Learning to eat a healthy diet and maintain an ideal weight are still important factors in managing PCOS and being healthy during pregnancy and beyond.

Intrauterine Insemination (IUI)

IUI is more affordable than IVF, but has a lower success rate. During IUI, healthy sperm are placed inside the uterus during ovulation to increase the chance of fertilization. IUI is usually the first step of fertility treatments because it is non-invasive, so several cycles may be completed before your specialists recommend you try something else. Sometimes insurance companies actually require that you try a few rounds of IUI before they will cover other treatments.

In vitro Fertilization

In vitro fertilization (IVF) is when a mature egg is retrieved from your ovaries before being fertilized with sperm in a laboratory. The embryos are then implanted in your uterus to develop. An IVF cycle takes several weeks to complete, and requires frequent blood tests and daily hormone injections to encourage the embryo to implant and grow. IVF has a high success rate, and gives you more control over having multiples because the doctor can implant just one embryo at a time.

Gamete Intrafallopian Transfer

Gamete Intrafallopian Transfer (GIFT) is when an egg is taken from your uterus and placed in your fallopian tube, along with sperm to fertilize it. This is somewhat similar to IVF, except with IVF, the fertilization takes place in a lab before the embryo is inserted into your uterus.

It takes about six weeks to complete a cycle of GIFT. You will take fertility drugs until the doctor sees a viable egg. The egg is harvested, mixed with sperm, and then inserted into the fallopian tube.

With advances in IVF, GIFT is not being used as frequently as it used to be, since the woman has to undergo a procedure to have her egg removed, then another to have it put into her fallopian tube.

Surgical Options

If medications and assisted reproductive technologies are not successful, your specialist might suggest trying various surgical fertility procedures available for women with PCOS. With assisted reproductive technologies being so successful, it is rare that you will get to this point, but it is a good idea to know your options.

Ovarian Drilling

Ovarian drilling is a surgery that entails the doctor using lasers or a fine needle to make a few holes in the surface of your ovary. This surgery works to revitalize ovulation and changes your hormone levels, but it is only effective for six to eight months. Studies have shown that over half of the women who have ovarian drilling get pregnant within a year after the surgery.

In rare cases, ovarian drilling may cause women with PCOS to have lower ovarian reserves. This means that, if it takes them many attempts to get pregnant, they might need an egg donor.

Hysteroscopic Surgery

A hysteroscopic surgery is a mildly invasive operation that removes or corrects any uterine abnormalities to help improve your chances of getting pregnant. The surgeon looks at the shape of the uterus, which can be corrected. They will look for fibroids or polyps, which can be removed. The surgeon will also check the lining of the uterus and find the openings to the fallopian tubes. If the lining does not look optimal for a pregnancy, or if the fallopian tubes are not opening properly, then further action will be taken from there.

Tubal Surgery

If your fallopian tubes are filled with fluid or blocked, you may need tubal surgery to dilate a tube or create a new opening. Tubal surgery is rare because pregnancy rates are higher with IVF, but your doctor might recommend tubal surgery if they feel it will help you conceive.

Chapter 7:

Managing Your PCOS Symptoms

Losing weight, exercising, and making major lifestyle changes can help you manage PCOS and get pregnant, but there are other conditions that often cannot be managed just by lifestyle changes. While some of these symptoms can be improved by changes in your lifestyle that influence your hormone levels, you might not want to wait long enough to see changes. These are additional methods for ways you might want to manage PCOS symptoms that cannot be easily changed otherwise.

Hirsutism

There are many ways to remove unwanted hair caused by hirsutism. If you are taking medication for other PCOS symptoms, some side effects might positively impact your hirsutism. These include birth control pills and spironolactone, which balance your hormones and prevent excessive androgen production. Eflornithine is a prescription cream that can slow the growth of your facial hair growth.

Temporary hair removal methods can be found in most drug stores or beauty supply stores. You can shave the hair using standard razors or more delicate single blade razors intended for women to use on facial hair. You can pluck the hairs, which tear it from its follicle, but this method can be time-intensive for larger patches of hair, and can irritate your skin.

Hair removal creams work to break down the keratin and dissolve the hair. Not all creams are safe to be used on your face, and some may cause skin irritation, so test a small area before using a lot of it. If you have acne along with hirsutism, using a cream might cause your acne to flare up as well. Waxing is another option, but it is only safe on certain areas of the body, and might still cause irritation or even infection.

If you do not want to remove the hair, just have it be less noticeable, then you can try bleaching it. Bleach is a strong chemical so you will want to do it only on small patches of skin, and stop usage if your skin gets irritated or damaged.

Cosmetic hair removal is permanent and takes several sessions to complete. If you want to try cosmetic hair removal, talk to your doctor and make sure to get a referral. Some insurances cover permanent hair removal, so you might want to look into your options.

Electrolysis is a method that destroys the hair's growth center with chemical energy. A fine probe is inserted into the hair follicle and then the hair is removed with tweezers. Electrolysis can be used on many different areas of the body, like the face, legs, breasts, and abdomen. Side effects from electrolysis are rare, unless it is a slight reddening of the skin that is only temporary.

Laser hair removal can be used on larger areas of the body than electrolysis, but the long-term effectiveness is not as positive as electrolysis. Women who get laser hair removal typically see some regrowth after a few months because the process mostly damages hair follicles instead of destroying them.

Hair Loss

Unfortunately, the hair that you have lost as a side effect of PCOS will not grow back naturally, but there are treatments available that might stimulate the growth of new hair. Birth control pills and spironolactone are medications prescribed to manage other PCOS symptoms. They lower your body's androgen and testosterone levels to prevent future hair loss.

Minoxidil is the only treatment for female pattern baldness that has been approved by the Food and Drug Administration (FDA). It is a topical solution that you apply to your scalp every day to promote hair growth.

Women with PCOS who have used Minoxidil say that their hair grew back even thicker than it had been before.

Finasteride and Dutasteride are additional hair loss treatments, but they only have FDA-approval for treating male pattern hair loss. Some doctors prescribe them to women with PCOS, but there is not much research available on how effective they are.

Whether you are using hair growth treatments and waiting to see a difference, or if you prefer to not use any chemical solutions, there are clever ways to disguise your hair loss. If your part is getting wider, you can start parting your hair on other areas of your head. This will give you a new style while helping disguise your hair loss. You could also try bangs, and get them cut from hair farther back on your head.

For thinning hair, you could wear a partial wig, also called a wig fall. These are worn on top of your existing hair to add volume without damaging your hair with glue. You could also change your hairstyle by getting your hair cut shorter with layers to add volume and make your hair look full. You can use volumizing hair products to help.

If you have bald patches, you can change your hairstyle to cover the bald parts. Low ponytails and top knots are cute stylish ways you can hide bald spots. You could also position a headband on the right spot, or tie a cute scarf around your hair. Partial wigs and wig falls work well to cover bald spots too, just as they do for thinning hair.

If you are not getting satisfactory results from any of the above methods, you could consider a hair transplant. This is a surgical procedure that takes hair from elsewhere on your body and implants it on your scalp. These transplants are incredibly expensive, and are considered cosmetic so most insurances will not cover the cost.

Acne

Women with PCOS can develop cystic hormonal acne, which is more painful than standard acne. Acne is caused by hormones, stress, bacteria, and skin type, so women with PCOS already have elevated internal issues making them susceptible to cystic acne.

To treat this type of acne, you should focus on treating the root cause of PCOS instead of the acne itself. Common over-the-counter acne treatments are made with benzoyl peroxide and salicylic acid, which only attack acne from the skin level. Hormonal acne is caused by your hormone levels more than bacteria or dirt irritating your skin, so it needs to be treated from the inside.

Birth control pills and spironolactone are used to manage other PCOS symptoms, and since they balance your hormones internally, they might help alleviate your hormonal acne as well. However, this is not what the pills are made for, it is just a positive side effect.

Eating a healthy diet will also help balance your hormones and regulate your body's functions in ways that can benefit your acne. Exercise is another good way to improve your hormone levels. When you get sweaty from exercising, be sure to be extra diligent with your skincare routine. You should already be washing your face every morning and evening, but definitely wash it after sweating. Do not scrub your skin, because this irritates it and can cause your acne to flare. Using your fingers to apply a nonabrasive cleanser is better for your skin, because your touch is gentler than a washcloth or sponge. You can even just splash your skin with lukewarm water when you are done, instead of using a washcloth to wipe off the cleanser.

To keep your skin healthy, you should never touch, squeeze, or pop your pimples. It does not help them go away, it only spreads the bacteria and makes things worse. It is hard to be patient when your skin feels so painful, but treating your skin right will pay off in the long run. You also should avoid tanning beds and extreme exposure to the sun, though moderate amounts of vitamin D from the sun can help heal your skin.

Other Skin Issues

Among all the other issues we have discussed, insulin resistance can also cause dark patches of skin on women with PCOS. These dark patches might be found in your armpits, groin area, on your neck, elbows, knees, knuckles and even your lips. As you work to balance your diet and get your insulin levels under control most of these dark patches will disappear on their own. Zinc supplements and other nutrients that balance your hormones can also cause these spots to fade.

While you are waiting for your levels to even out internally, there are some external options to make your skin look smoother. You can use skin brightening serums to even out your skin color, or match a darker foundation to the spots on your face and use that to blend them in. You can also exfoliate your skin often, because this removes dead skin cells to help lighten your skin. Since exfoliation is a gritty process, make sure to hydrate your skin afterwards. Coconut oil is an ideal choice because it has healthy fats that will help heal, rejuvenate, and moisturize your skin.

If none of these options are helping to eliminate your dark spots, ask your dermatologist if a cosmetic treatment can help. Dermabrasion is like a surgical exfoliation where a dermatologist or plastic surgeon uses a rotating device to scrape off the outer layers of skin. It is usually done on facial skin, and in addition to lightening your dark spots, it can treat your fine lines, acne scars, and even out the texture of your skin.

Laser therapy is a way of removing the top layer of discolored skin so that new, lighter skin cells can form. Laser therapy can irritate acne, so if you have both acne and dark spots, this might not be an effective treatment for you. You should also talk to your doctor before starting treatment, because it can interfere with some supplements and medications that affect blood clotting.

PCOS can also cause skin tags. These are small flaps or lumps of skin that are harmless and do not cause any pain. They typically form in places where your skin rubs together, like in your armpits, on your neck, on your eyelids, in your groin area, or under your breasts. They can be skin-colored or red, so you might not like how they look and want to remove them. They can also be in places on your body where they constantly get caught in your hair, jewelry, or get rubbed by your clothes, so you might want them removed just for peace of mind.

The best way to eliminate skin tags is through cryotherapy. This is a method of using freezing or near-freezing liquid nitrogen to remove the skin tag. It will fall off ten to fourteen days after being frozen. This treatment can cause some redness or irritation to the surrounding skin, but otherwise is not harmful or painful.

Mental Health Issues

Dealing with PCOS and the struggle to get diagnosed and manage symptoms is a massive undertaking, so it is no surprise that many women with PCOS suffer from depression. Depressive features, anxiety, poor body image issues and negative self-esteem are associated comorbidities that make PCOS more than just a physical disorder, but sometimes doctors do not think about this when they are treating you. Do not be afraid to advocate for yourself and your mental health by asking for medications to balance your hormones or referrals for talk therapists.

Before you take medication or go to therapy, be sure you are putting in all the work you can to help yourself. I cannot stress enough how important it is for your whole-body health to eat right and exercise. It might seem like a superficial thing, but I am not talking at all about how losing weight makes you look. I am purely talking about how being healthy and active makes you feel. It will give you energy and get your heart and blood pumping and you will feel much better than if you stayed on the couch wallowing.

That being said, there are medications and supplements you can take to improve your mental health, and you should not feel ashamed for taking them. Mental health is just as important as physical health, and they actually impact each other in a cycle. So you, along with your doctor, need to make the decisions about what treatments are the best to improve your mental health.

Your doctor knows you and has been on this PCOS journey with you, so they will know that the best way to improve your depression is to treat the underlying cause. This might mean they prescribe medications to balance your insulin and hormones, like metformin and birth control pills.

Antidepressants are usually prescribed to treat depression, but some cause weight gain and can mess up your blood glucose levels, so they are not the best option for women with PCOS. However, if the other medications do not seem to work, your doctor might analyze your glucose levels and weight history and prescribe antidepressants. At some point, you have to decide what you are willing to live with when it comes to the balance of mental health and physical health.

Whether you do it instead of or in addition to medication, talk therapy is an effective treatment for depression. Also called counseling, this option gives you an outlet for your thoughts and feelings, and a licensed professional can help you figure out possible solutions for what you are going through.

Cognitive behavioral therapy is a psychological treatment that is effective for treating a range of problems including depression and anxiety disorders. It can help you identify and change any ingrained negative thinking patterns and teach you coping strategies so you can get past them. The best thing about cognitive behavioral therapy is that, once you learn it, you can practice it on yourself, anytime, anywhere.

Emotional Health Care

Emotional problems are common in women with PCOS. The symptoms of PCOS can cause a lot of physical pain, which in turn affects you emotionally. Outward symptoms of PCOS like hirsutism, acne, and weight gain can also make you feel depressed or send your self-esteem plummeting. Suffering from infertility is enough to send anyone into a depressive spiral, but if you add all of these other symptoms into the mix, it can seem impossible to get out of bed some days.

You have learned all about eating a healthy diet and you know how that can benefit your body physically, but it can also improve your emotional well-being. Eating a balanced diet that gives your body all of the nutrients it needs will help keep you mentally balanced. Eating healthy food makes your body feel good, and in turn your mind and emotional well-being will also feel good. Once your healthy eating starts to pay off with weight loss, your emotional health will soar through the roof as your self-confidence improves.

Emotional well-being can also impact your diet. If you are feeling bad, you are more likely to make bad food choices in the name of comfort, or just wanting to eat something because there is nothing else you feel like doing. If you feel stable emotionally, you will be able to think logically about your food choices and continue making good decisions.

Taking care of yourself and all of your PCOS symptoms is a lot, and it is hard to do day in and day out. But remember that you have a team of people helping you. If you feel like you are struggling emotionally, talk to your doctor, gynecologist, or other specialists. They will understand how you are feeling and why. If they cannot help you, they can recommend someone who can. Talk therapy can be a huge help for all women, whether they have PCOS or not. So know that you do not have to carry this weight alone, and do not be afraid to seek help.

Hopefully you also have a supportive team of friends and family helping you on this journey. Sometimes just talking to someone who knows what you are going through can really help. You do not even have to talk about what you are feeling at that moment; you can use the friend as an escape from your own life and just forget your troubles for a bit. They know what you are going through, and that can be enough.

If you do not have anyone supportive around you who can help you get through the tough times, find someone or tell someone. It might seem easier to keep your condition to yourself. You might feel like it is too personal, and you like to be private. Or you might not want to burden your loved ones with the details of your condition. But just think about telling someone close to you. They might become a strong pillar you can depend on to help you through this journey.

If you want to stay private and keep your health concerns personal, you can do that! You do not have to spill your guts to friends or family to find support. Join forums and message boards for women diagnosed with PCOS, because you know they will understand what you are going through. Ask your doctors and specialists if they know of any in-person support groups you could attend to find some local friends who know what it is like.

Conclusion

Now that you have a solid foundation of understanding PCOS and how you can manage the symptoms, you should feel empowered to advocate for yourself. All of the knowledge in this book has given you will help you improve your diet, easily add physical activity into your daily life, and work to naturally balance your hormone levels.

Information about medications and medical options to alleviate your PCOS symptoms, manage the related complications, and increase your fertility has shown you that it is possible to live an enjoyable life, even though you have been diagnosed with an incurable condition. I want to wish you well and leave you with some inspirational success stories.

Linda has had PCOS since she was eleven, but she was not diagnosed until she was twenty-one. The two years after diagnosis were her worst—she gained a lot of weight, coming in at over three hundred pounds. She was relieved to finally have a name for her condition, but she had no clue how to manage it. She tried exercising, but could not lose weight. She was on the birth control pill to regulate her periods, but that was all it did for her.

On a whim, Linda tried a keto diet when she turned twenty-four. She was amazed at how much energy she had all day, and how she could actually tell she was losing weight due to the combination of a balanced diet and exercise. She considers her PCOS in remission because she has not had a symptom in over five years. The best part is, Linda is pregnant!

Linda recommends trying a keto diet if you cannot find anything that works for you. Eliminating carbs and sugar were the one thing that made all the difference for her. But she warns against going cold turkey and cutting out carbs completely, because you are more likely to backslide into your old eating habits. Instead, change your diet slowly, eating fewer and fewer carbs and sugar until your body adjusts and your tastes change.

Kallie has always been athletic, but she had to work really hard to maintain her weight so that she could compete in her weight class. She was frustrated that it took so much exercise and calorie-counting to keep her body from becoming overweight, when the work she was doing should have kept her lean while building up her muscles. She finally got fed up with the situation and went to a doctor, who diagnosed her with PCOS.

Kallie had never researched the condition; she thought her period was irregular due to her athleticism. She figured something was off with her body since she could not lose weight, but she never would have guessed her insulin levels were the culprit. In fact, her doctor told her she was prediabetic. As someone who always ate healthy foods, she was shocked. It was then that Kallie realized the standard food pyramid is not right for everyone.

Kallie now considers herself "carbohydrate intolerant" and eats a moderate amount of protein, a lot of non-starchy vegetables, and a lot of healthy fats. Over time she has found that she can eat a small amount of carbohydrates if they come from beans or lentils instead of pasta and bread. And she has completely stopped counting calories.

Stephanie was diagnosed with PCOS at nineteen and was told she probably would not be able to have a baby. She kind of shrugged it off because she was only nineteen! She did not even have a boyfriend, so a baby was the farthest thing from her mind. Stephanie did not have a period throughout her twenties, but she was focusing on her career so it barely even registered.

Once she hit her thirties, Stephanie was ready to start a family, but was having trouble getting pregnant. She started researching infertility until the light bulb went off in her head—oh right, PCOS. She focused her research specifically on infertility in women with PCOS and made all the necessary diet, exercise, and lifestyle changes. Within a year, she was getting a regular period. After a few cycles, she was able to pinpoint her ovulation days, and became pregnant naturally, even though she had PCOS and was in her mid-thirties! Needless to say, Stephanie was shocked. But she loved being a mother, and wanted to try for a second child. She was used to managing her PCOS symptoms by this time, but was still surprised when she got pregnant quickly and easily.

Stephanie knows that this story will not happen for everyone, but she says having hope is important. After all, her doctor told her she would probably not be able to have a baby, and she did not have periods for a decade, but still got pregnant naturally after managing her PCOS. If that is not an inspirational story, I do not know what is!

If you enjoyed this book, please leave a review on Amazon. This will help others who are suffering from PCOS know they can find quality information, research, and support in this book. Thank you, and best of luck!

References

30 Interesting Facts About PCOS. (2017, September 1). PCOS Nutrition Center.

    http://www.pcosnutrition.com/facts/

Endometrial Cancer. (n.d.). Www.Cancer.org.

    https://www.cancer.org/cancer/endometrial-cancer.html

Ovarian Cysts. (n.d.). Medlineplus.Gov. https://medlineplus.gov/ovariancysts.html

Patel, V., Menezes, H., Menezes, C., Bouwer, S., Bostick-Smith, C. A., & Speelman, D. L.

    (2020). Regular Mindful Yoga Practice as a Method to Improve Androgen Levels

    in Women With Polycystic Ovary Syndrome: A Randomized, Controlled Trial.

    The Journal of the American Osteopathic Association.

    https://doi.org/10.7556/jaoa.2020.050

Polycystic Ovary Syndrome (PCOS). (2019).

    https://www.hopkinsmedicine.org/health/conditions-and-diseases/polycystic-ov

ary-syndrome-pcos

Polycystic ovary syndrome | Womenshealth.gov. (2019, April). Womenshealth.Gov.

https://www.womenshealth.gov/a-z-topics/polycystic-ovary-syndrome

Progestin treatment for polycystic ovarian syndrome may reduce pregnancy chances.

(2015, August 31). National Institutes of Health (NIH).

https://www.nih.gov/news-events/news-releases/progestin-treatment-polycystic

-ovarian-syndrome-may-reduce-pregnancy-chances

Rao, M., Broughton, K. S., & LeMieux, M. J. (2020). Cross-sectional Study on the

Knowledge and Prevalence of PCOS at a Multiethnic University. *Progress in*

Preventive Medicine, 5(2), e0028.

https://doi.org/10.1097/pp9.0000000000000028

Shamasbi, S. G., Ghanbari-Homayi, S., & Mirghafourvand, M. (2019). The effect of

probiotics, prebiotics, and synbiotics on hormonal and inflammatory indices in